Ear, Nose, and Throat Conditions

Editor

DANIEL D. SMEAK

VETERINARY CLINICS
OF NORTH AMERICA:
SMALL ANIMAL PRACTICE

www.vetsmall.theclinics.com

July 2016 • Volume 46 • Number 4

ELSEVIER

1600 John F. Kennedy Boulevard • Suite 1800 • Philadelphia, Pennsylvania, 19103-2899
http://www.vetsmall.theclinics.com

VETERINARY CLINICS OF NORTH AMERICA: SMALL ANIMAL PRACTICE Volume 46, Number 4
July 2016 ISSN 0195-5616, ISBN-13: 978-0-323-44859-8

Editor: Patrick Manley
Developmental Editor: Meredith Clinton

Veterinary Clinics of North America: Small Animal Practice (ISSN 0195-5616) is published bimonthly by Elsevier Inc., 360 Park Avenue South, New York, NY 10010-1710. Months of issue are January, March, May, July, September, and November. Business and Editorial Offices: 1600 John F. Kennedy Blvd., Ste. 1800, Philadelphia, PA 19103-2899. Customer Service Office: 3251 Riverport Lane, Maryland Heights, MO 63043. Periodicals postage paid at New York, NY and additional mailing offices. Subscription prices are $310.00 per year (domestic individuals), $564.00 per year (domestic institutions), $100.00 per year (domestic students/residents), $410.00 per year (Canadian individuals), $701.00 per year (Canadian institutions), $455.00 per year (international individuals), $701.00 per year (international institutions), and $220.00 per year (international and Canadian students/residents). To receive student/resident rate, orders must be accompanied by name of affiliated institution, date of term, and the *signature* of program/residency coordinator on institution letterhead. Orders will be billed at individual rate until proof of status is received. Foreign air speed delivery is included in all *Clinics* subscription prices. All prices are subject to change without notice. **POSTMASTER:** Send address changes to *Veterinary Clinics of North America: Small Animal Practice*, Elsevier Health Sciences Division, Subscription Customer Service, 3251 Riverport Lane, Maryland Heights, MO 63043. Customer Service (orders, claims, online, change of address): Elsevier Periodicals Customer Service, Elsevier Health Sciences Division Subscription **Customer Service 3251 Riverport Lane Maryland Heights, MO 63043. Tel: 1-800-654-2452 (U.S. and Canada); 314-447-8871 (outside U.S. and Canada). Fax: 314-447-8029. E-mail: journalscustomerservice-usa@elsevier.com (for print support); journalsonlinesupport-usa@elsevier.com (for online support).**

Reprints. For copies of 100 or more of articles in this publication, please contact the Commercial Reprints Department, Elsevier Inc., 360 Park Avenue South, New York, NY 10010-1710. Tel.: 212-633-3874; Fax: 212-633-3820; E-mail: reprints@elsevier.com.

Veterinary Clinics of North America: Small Animal Practice is also published in Japanese by Inter Zoo Publishing Co., Ltd., Aoyama Crystal-Bldg 5F, 3-5-12 Kitaaoyama, Minato-ku, Tokyo 107-0061, Japan.

Veterinary Clinics of North America: Small Animal Practice is covered in *Current Contents/Agriculture, Biology and Environmental Sciences, Science Citation Index, ASCA, MEDLINE/PubMed (Index Medicus), Excerpta Medica,* and *BIOSIS*.

Contributors

EDITOR

DANIEL D. SMEAK, DVM
Diplomate, American College of Veterinary Surgeons; Professor and Chief of Small Animal Surgery, and Dental and Oral Surgery, Department of Veterinary Clinical Sciences, College of Veterinary Medicine and Biomedical Sciences; James L. Voss Veterinary Teaching Hospital, Colorado State University, Fort Collins, Colorado

AUTHORS

BOAZ ARZI, DVM
Diplomate, American Veterinary Dental College; Diplomate, European Veterinary Dental College; Assistant Professor of Dentistry and Oral Surgery, Department of Surgical and Radiological Sciences, School of Veterinary Medicine, University of California - Davis, Davis, California

ALLYSON C. BERENT, DVM
Diplomate, American College of Veterinary Internal Medicine; Director, Interventional Endoscopy Services, Department of Interventional Radiology and Endoscopy, Internal Medicine, The Animal Medical Center, New York, New York

DANIEL ALVIN DEGNER, DVM
Diplomate of the American College of Veterinary Surgeons; Staff Surgeon, Animal Surgical Center of Michigan, Flint, Michigan

GILLES DUPRÉ, Univ Prof Dr Med Vet
Diplomate, European College of Veterinary Surgery; Head, Department of Small Animal Surgery and Equine, Vetmeduni Vienna, Veterinary Medicine University, Vienna, Austria

NADINE FIANI, BVSc
Diplomate, American Veterinary Dental College; Clinical Assistant Professor of Dentistry and Oral Surgery, Department of Clinical Sciences, College of Veterinary Medicine, Cornell University, Ithaca, New York

VALENTINA GRECI, DVM, PhD
Internal Medicine and Endoscopy, Ospedale Veterinario Gregorio VII, Roma, Italia

DOROTHEE HEIDENREICH, Dr Med Vet
ECVS Board-eligible Small Animal Surgeon, Department of Small Animal Surgery and Equine, Vetmeduni Vienna, Veterinary Medicine University, Vienna, Austria

CATRIONA MacPHAIL, DVM, PhD
Diplomate, American College of Veterinary Surgeons; Associate Professor, Department of Clinical Sciences, College of Veterinary Medicine and Biomedical Sciences, Colorado State University, Fort Collins, Colorado

ERIC MONNET, DVM, PhD
Diplomate, American College of Veterinary Surgeons; Diplomate, European College
of Veterinary Surgeons; Department of Clinical Sciences, College of Veterinary Medicine
and Biomedical Sciences, Colorado State University, Fort Collins, Colorado

CARLO MARIA MORTELLARO, DVM
Professor, Division of Small Animal Surgery, Department of Veterinary Medicine, Facoltà
di Medicina Veterinaria, Università degli Studi di Milano, Milano, Italia

MARIJE RISSELADA, DVM, PhD
Diplomate, European College of Veterinary Surgery; Diplomate, American College of
Veterinary Surgery - Small Animals; Assistant Professor, Small Animal Soft Tissue and
Oncologic Surgery, Department of Clinical Sciences, College of Veterinary Medicine,
North Carolina State University, Raleigh, North Carolina

DANIEL D. SMEAK, DVM
Diplomate, American College of Veterinary Surgeons; Professor and Chief of Small Animal
Surgery, and Dental and Oral Surgery, Department of Veterinary Clinical Sciences,
College of Veterinary Medicine and Biomedical Sciences; James L. Voss Veterinary
Teaching Hospital, Colorado State University, Fort Collins, Colorado

FRANK J.M. VERSTRAETE, DrMedVet, MMedVet
Diplomate, American Veterinary Dental College; Diplomate, European College of
Veterinary Surgeons; Diplomate, European Veterinary Dental College; Professor of
Dentistry and Oral Surgery, Department of Surgical and Radiological Sciences,
School of Veterinary Medicine, University of California - Davis, Davis, California

ALYSSA MARIE WEEDEN, DVM
Small Animal Medicine and Surgery Intern, Animal Surgical Center of Michigan, Flint,
Michigan

DEANNA R. WORLEY, DVM
Diplomate, American College of Veterinary Surgeons - Small Animal; American College of
Veterinary Surgeons Founding Fellow, Surgical Oncology; Associate Professor, Surgical
Oncology, Department of Clinical Sciences and Flint Animal Cancer Center, Colorado
State University, Fort Collins, Colorado

Contents

> Persistent deep infection originating from remnants of an incompletely excised ear canal, or epithelium and debris left in the osseous ear canal or tympanic cavity after surgery total ear canal ablation and lateral bulla osteotomy can be debilitating. Clinical signs including pain elicited on deep palpation over the affected bulla or when opening the mouth, or draining sinuses may be delayed months to years. Localization of the nidus via CT imaging is important for surgical planning. Although antibiotic therapy usually reduces or eliminates the clinical signs of deep infection, relapses are common. Surgery more consistently results in permanent resolution.

> Surgical intervention of aural cholesteatomas in dogs can be curative. Imaging findings include a soft tissue density in the middle ear and destruction of the bone of the bulla with characteristics of an aggressive lesion. Dogs with early stage disease have a better outcome than those with chronic disease, temporal bone involvement and neurologic signs. Dogs with recurrent disease can be reoperated or managed medically with long-term resolution or palliation of clinical signs.

> Ear disease, such as otitis externa, resulting in aggressive head shaking or ear scratching, is the most common cause of the development of aural hematomas in dogs and cats. An underlying immunologic cause has also been proposed to explain cartilage and blood vessel fragility. Numerous options exist for management of aural hematomas, from medical management alone with corticosteroids, to simple hematoma centesis, to surgical intervention. Because this condition is usually secondary to another disease process, regardless of mode of treatment, likelihood of recurrence is low if the underlying condition is managed properly.

> Feline inflammatory polyps are the most common nonneoplastic lesion of ear and nasopharynx in cats. Minimally invasive techniques for polyp

removal, such as traction avulsion combined with curettage of the tympanic cavity and per-endoscopic transtympanic traction, have been successful for long-term resolution. Feline nasal hamartomas are benign lesions of the nasopharynx, and most have a good prognosis after surgical removal. Canine aural and nasopharyngeal inflammatory polyps are rare and have a similar clinical presentation as cats with these lesions. In dogs, it is important to achieve an accurate histologic diagnosis of these masses before appropriate surgical treatment can be planned.

Clefts of the primary palate in the dog are uncommon, and their repair can be challenging. The aims of this article are to provide information regarding pathogenesis and convey practical information for the repair of these defects.

Choanal atresia is rare in small animal veterinary medicine, and most cases are misdiagnosed and are actually a nasopharyngeal stenosis (NPS), which is frustrating to treat because of the high recurrence rates encountered after surgical intervention. Minimally invasive treatment options like balloon dilation (BD), metallic stent placement (MS), or covered metallic stent (CMS) placement have been met with success but are associated with various complications that must be considered. The most common complication with BD alone is stenosis recurrence. The most common complications encountered with MS placement is tissue ingrowth, chronic infections and the development of an oronasal fistula. The most common complications with a CMS is chronic infections and the development of an oronasal fistula, but stricture recurrence is avoided.

Animals presenting with brachycephalic syndrome suffer from multilevel obstruction of the airways as well as secondary structural collapse. Stenotic nares, aberrant turbinates, nasopharyngeal collapse, soft palate elongation and hyperplasia, laryngeal collapse, and left bronchus collapse are being described as the most common associated anomalies. Rhinoplasty and palatoplasty as well as newer surgical techniques and postoperative care strategies have resulted in significant improvement of the prognosis even in middle-aged dogs.

VETERINARY CLINICS OF NORTH AMERICA: SMALL ANIMAL PRACTICE

RELATED INTEREST

Veterinary Clinics of North America: Exotic Animal Practice
May 2016, Volume 19, Issue 2
Emergency and Critical Care
Margaret Fordham and Brian Roberts, *Editors*

THE CLINICS ARE NOW AVAILABLE ONLINE!
Access your subscription at:
www.theclinics.com

Preface

Ear, Nose, and Throat Conditions: Purpose and Acknowledgment

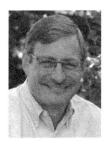

Daniel D. Smeak, DVM
Editor

During the early stages of my surgical residency at The Ohio State University, I recognized that we often learn the most about a surgical condition through the process of understanding and treating complications arising from the surgical procedures we perform. I began to realize that many of the complications we encounter can be prevented by a thorough understanding of the pathophysiology of the surgical disease, and incorporating core surgical principles and a thorough understanding of the regional anatomy into the planning and execution of the procedure. As I progressed through my residency training, I was alarmed at the number of complications we were encountering following total ear canal ablation. Many of these complications caused patient morbidity far worse than the condition that the surgery was designed to treat. I could find little information about proper management of these complications, and I began to question the way we surgeons approached end-stage inflammatory ear disease. This search prompted the first publication of my career, a retrospective study documenting an embarrassing number of complications after total ear canal ablation, particularly acute and chronic wound infection. At first we believed that poor drainage of the surgical site and tympanic bulla was the main reason for the high infection risk. Incorporation of various wound drainage techniques following this procedure did not significantly reduce infections, and in some cases caused other problems. As advanced imaging emerged, we began to pay particular attention to the middle ear changes involved in chronic end-stage inflammatory ear disease. We have since made significant advances in surgical exposure of the tympanic bulla by aggressive subtotal lateral bulla osteotomy, allowing us the ability to thoroughly debride migrating epithelium and debris within bulla while preserving important regional neurologic and vascular structures. It is now expected that nearly all our patients affected by end-stage ear disease will enjoy long-term relief after surgery. It is

Vet Clin Small Anim 46 (2016) ix–x
http://dx.doi.org/10.1016/j.cvsm.2016.03.001
0195-5616/16/$ – see front matter © 2016 Published by Elsevier Inc.

these breakthroughs in our understanding of surgical diseases, and our continued desire to improve our diagnostic and surgical techniques, that keeps me passionate and engaged in my general surgical practice and academic career.

Surgical conditions affecting the ear, nose, and throat in dogs and cats are some of the more common diseases presenting to small animal practitioners and surgical specialists alike. I have chosen a number of select topics to cover in this issue with new and emerging diagnostic and therapeutic options for ear, nose, and throat conditions. The topics are organized starting with clinical updates surrounding the ear of dogs and cats, and then surgical conditions affecting the nose and nasopharynx, and finally the larynx. I have asked authors whenever possible to include detailed current information about the pathophysiology of their surgical topic, and to incorporate pertinent core surgical principles, regional anatomy, and complications when describing their surgical treatment options and recommendations. In the first article of this issue, I examine why deep infections occur after total ear canal ablation and how to effectively diagnose and manage these deep abscesses and chronic fistulas. Dr Risselada examines cholesteatomas, debilitating expansile growths within the tympanic bulla, and why this disease continues to be a demanding surgical condition to successfully treat. New and traditional methods to treat auricular hematomas are described by Dr MacPhail. Drs Greci and Mortellaro offer updated information about treatment of otic and nasopharyngeal polyps seen commonly in cats, and more rarely in dogs. Newer surgical techniques for reconstruction of congenital nose, palate, and lip disorders are covered by Drs Fiani, Verstraete, and Arzi. Drs Weeden and Degner illustrate an array of standard and novel surgical approaches to the nasal cavity and sinuses. Dr Worley describes our current understanding of nose and nasal planum neoplasia, and how to reconstruct facial defects after aggressive surgical excision. Dr Berent explains her current recommendations for treatment of one of the most challenging disease conditions encountered in my practice, nasopharyngeal stenosis. Dr Dupre and Heidenreich offer novel surgical options for treatment of dogs afflicted with brachycephalic syndrome. Finally, Dr Monnet provides an update on current treatment recommendations for laryngeal paralysis in dogs. I thank all of these exceptional authors for sharing their valuable experience, expertise, and scientific contribution to this issue. I also wish to recognize these busy clinicians for their extra time and effort in preparing well-written articles on time!

Finally, I want to personally thank Patrick Manley and Meredith Clinton, from Elsevier, for the opportunity to be the guest editor of this issue of *Veterinary Clinics of North America: Small Animal Practice*. My hope is that this collection of articles on ear, nose, and throat conditions will help update veterinarians so they can offer the very best recommendations and latest treatment options for their patients.

Daniel D. Smeak, DVM
Department of Veterinary Clinical Sciences
College of Veterinary Medicine and
Biomedical Sciences
James L. Voss Veterinary Teaching Hospital
300 West Drake Road
Fort Collins, CO 85023-1026, USA

E-mail address:
dan.smeak@colostate.edu

Treatment of Persistent Deep Infection After Total Ear Canal Ablation and Lateral Bulla Osteotomy

CrossMark

Daniel D. Smeak, DVM

KEYWORDS

- Surgery • Dog • Ear canal ablation • Deep infection

KEY POINTS

- Deep infection following total ear canal ablation (TECA) and lateral bulla osteotomy (LBO) is thought to originate from remnants of an incompletely excised ear canal, or epithelium and debris left in the osseous ear canal or tympanic cavity after surgery.
- Clinical signs may be delayed months to years following TECA-LBO.
- Facial swelling or fistula formation in the region of the original incision, pain elicited on deep palpation over the affected bulla or when opening the mouth are clinical signs seen with deep infection.
- Dogs often respond to antibiotic therapy but recurrence of signs is common after therapy is withdrawn.
- Contrast CT often helps accurately locate the nidus of infection for surgical planning.

INTRODUCTION

Surgery is often recommended by veterinarians for small animals that present for what is referred to as end-stage otitis.[1] Although chronic deep-seated infection with ear canal epithelial hyperplasia, stenosis, and calcification is the most common end-stage ear condition seen by practitioners, unresponsive middle ear infection, cholesteatoma, neoplastic infiltration of the ear canal or middle ear, and severe trauma to the ear canal may also represent indications for surgical therapy.[1–7]

Total ear canal ablation (TECA) with lateral bulla osteotomy (LBO) remains the gold standard treatment of most end-stage ear diseases.[7,8] Up to 70% of dogs with chronic otitis externa have clinical evidence of otitis media,[9] so exploration of the tympanic

Disclosure Statement: The author has nothing to disclose.
Department of Veterinary Clinical Sciences, B207 Veterinary Teaching Hospital, College of Veterinary Medicine and Biomedical Sciences, Colorado State University, 300 West Drake Road, Fort Collins, CO 80523-1620, USA
E-mail address: dan.smeak@colostate.edu

cavity via LBO is now routinely performed with TECA.[10] As proliferative epithelial hyperplasia associated with chronic deep-seated ear canal infection expands into the ear canal, it out pouches or ruptures through the tympanic membrane, allowing abnormal epithelial migration into the tympanic bulla.[6] It is this displaced metaplastic epithelium that has been found as the nidus in many dogs afflicted with persistent deep infection following TECA.[11,12]

For the TECA-LBO to be successful long-term, the entire external ear canal is excised, and all debris and abnormal epithelium lining the external auditory meatus and tympanic cavity must be carefully and completely removed. This salvage procedure is demanding for even experienced surgeons because it requires tedious dissection to avoid important neurovascular structures that are not readily identified nor exposed during surgery.[13] In addition, a stenotic ear canal cannot be prepared well for aseptic surgery because debris and contaminants are not often completely removed during standard skin preparation and canal irrigation before surgery. During the surgical approach, because the affected ear canal is isolated and excised, and the lateral bulla wall is removed, substantial contamination of the exposed soft tissues is inevitable.[14]

Consequently, although recent retrospective studies have shown a decreasing trend in postoperative complications, especially acute wound infections following TECA-LBO, the procedure in the past has been associated with relatively high overall complication rates (up to 82% in some studies[15]), with most complications arising in the early postoperative period.[16] Incisional complications, such as prolonged wound drainage, incisional dehiscence, hematoma, seroma, and infection, have been reported to occur up to nearly one-third of TECA-LBO procedures.[16] Most of these wound complications are self-limiting and respond within days to weeks after antibiotic treatment and proper local wound management, including, in some cases, drainage, debridement, and even open wound management.[15,17]

When signs of infection persist or recur following local wound management, or signs appear well after the wound has healed successfully, deeper sources of infection should be investigated. The purposes of this article are to review the literature surrounding persistent or recurrent deep infection following TECA-LBO and to develop a diagnostic and therapeutic strategy for veterinarians who encounter this complication.

RATE OF DEEP INFECTION AFTER TOTAL EAR CANAL ABLATION AND LATERAL BULLA OSTEOTOMY

Deep infection manifested as chronic or recurrent fistulation adjacent to the TECA site, or abscessation deep to the subcutaneous tissue plane is reported to occur in up to 2% to 14% of dogs after TECA-LBO.[11,12,15,17–20] The actual rate may be even higher than this range because many retrospective studies do not provide long-term (more than 1 year) follow-up, and this complication may occur up to several years after TECA-LBO.[8,11,12,16] The risk of deep infection increases dramatically (up to 53%) when TECA-LBO is performed for dogs with end-stage ear disease and middle ear cholesteatomas because this expansile middle ear epithelial cyst is challenging to completely excise.[6] (Please see Risselada M: Diagnosis and Management of Cholesteatomas in Dogs, in this issue.)

The author could not find reports of chronic deep infection following TECA-LBO in cats.[21–23] Perhaps the reason for this difference is that TECA is performed more commonly for treatment of ear canal neoplasia in cats,[21,23] whereas in dogs chronic end-stage ear disease with deep seated bulla osteitis is by far the most common indication.[10] Cats have been reported to develop epithelial hyperplasia in response to chronic infection but migrated ear canal epithelium has not been reported during exploration of the middle ear in cats.[22] Furthermore, the ear canal in cats is shorter than most dogs, and this allows improved exposure when removing the ear canal and for exploration of the tympanic bulla. This may help surgeons avoid leaving a nidus of infection in this specie.

PATHOPHYSIOLOGY

A variety of sources of deep surgical site infection following TECA-LBO have been proposed but, in most cases documented in the literature, few have been substantiated. Osteomyelitis of the ossicles, tympanic bulla, and hyoid bone; poor drainage and inadequate removal of debris from the bulla at the time of surgery; inadequate drainage of the bulla from the auditory tube; parotid gland damage; and foreign material introduced at the time of surgery (eg, suture) have all been implicated as sources of deep infection after surgery.[1,17,20] In 1 report, retention of the tympanic membrane after TECA-LBO in normal experimental dogs resulted in accumulation of keratinized cellular debris, which could become a nidus of late abscessation in some dogs.[24] In nearly all reports of cases with recurrent deep infection that included detailed findings from exploration of the TECA-LBO site, 2 sources of infection have been confirmed: (1) epithelium and/or debris (hair, sebaceous material) found in the tympanic bulla or external auditory meatus, and/or (2) the horizontal ear canal was incompletely excised.[11,12,15,19,20] Epithelial remnants, including the tympanic membrane, produce keratin, glandular secretions, and even hair that can collect deep within the wound, and this material is thought to establish a persistent inflammatory focus.[11,12,24] The inflammatory focus welcomes secondary bacterial invasion, which persists unless the nidus is removed.[11,24]

It is now recognized that meticulous and complete removal of the ear canal and debris and secretory epithelium (with the tympanic membrane) from tympanic bulla and boney acoustic meatus are paramount to avoid debilitating consequences of deep infection developing after TECA-LBO.[11,12,24] The rate of wound complications, including chronic deep infection, has been not been shown to differ significantly whether or not wound drainage is provided after TECA-LBO.[2]

CLINICAL PRESENTATION

There does not seem to be a sex predilection for this complication. Of the 2 case series that specifically reported their findings about deep infection after TECA-LBO, one-third to one-half of the dogs were cocker spaniels.[11,12] This breed is most recognized for developing chronic proliferative otitis externa and, due to this predisposition, they are overrepresented in most retrospective studies of dogs undergoing TECA-LBO.[3]

Clinical signs suggesting a deep infection is forming may be delayed months to even years after surgery.

Dogs presented for treatment of para-aural fistulas from 1 month to 39 months (mean 10 months) after TECA-LBO in 1 study.[12] Likewise, other studies report fistula development ranging from 3 to 24 months after surgery.[15,17–20] Clinical signs of deep infection other than fistula formation, developed somewhat earlier at 1.5 months to 12 months (mean 5.5 months) in another case series report.[11] Perhaps signs of smoldering infection were overlooked by owners in some of the reports until overt fistula or abscesses developed months to years after surgery. In some dogs with mild intermittent clinical signs, it has been speculated that accumulated debris and fluid may be able to sporadically drain through the auditory tube from the deep regions of the wound.[24]

A variety of clinical signs of deep infection, some more subtle than others, have been reported. Clinical signs of deep infection may be obvious with single or multiple draining sinuses, or a ruptured abscess developing at or just rostroventral to the TECA site (**Fig. 1**). Nearly all dogs in 1 report resisted deep palpation over the ventral cervical area in the region of the affected bulla.[11] Painful swelling around the original incision region is common. Acute pain can be observed when opening the mouth in 20% to 45% of affected dogs.[11,12] A head tilt may develop on the affected side in some dogs, but no other neurologic signs have been reported other than those that were present before, or occurred from, the original TECA surgery. A minority of dogs present with a fever and an inflammatory leukogram.[11] Otherwise, expect no specific changes in cell blood counts and serum biochemical analyses. In the author's experience, anticipate some improvement in these clinical signs within days when affected dogs are treated with appropriate systemic antibiotics.

Owners should be made aware that early healing and successful recovery of their pet following TECA-LBO does not necessarily mean that late wound complications will not occur. Be sure to educate owners about clinical signs suggesting deep infection so early diagnosis and treatment can be undertaken. Once infection expands and becomes deep-seated, dogs may become recalcitrant to conservative medical management and require more aggressive surgical options.

DIFFERENTIAL DIAGNOSES

A history of TECA-LBO in a dog showing the aforementioned clinical signs should place deep infection high on the list of differential diagnoses. However, late onset clinical signs developing after TECA-LBO are not necessarily pathognomonic for deep infection related to the surgery. Other conditions that might appear include a deeply imbedded foreign body such as a grass awn or stick that penetrated the mouth or cervical area. Neoplastic conditions involving the temporal-mandibular joint, or surrounding structures, such as salivary or tonsillar tumors, may also mimic this condition. Severe sialadenitis or lymph node abscessation can also present with similar clinical signs. Thorough physical examination of the patient, with careful examination of the oral cavity and throat, are important to help differentiate these conditions from deep infection related to TECA-LBO. Progressive or multiple cranial nerve deficits or late

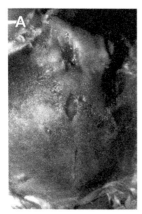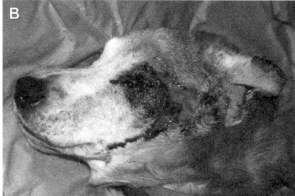

Fig. 1. (*A*) External appearance of a dog with a deep abscess under the original TECA incision. (*B*) A dog with multiple fistulas originating from a remnant of the horizontal ear canal after TECA.

onset Horner syndrome signs indicate a more aggressive disease process, such as neoplasia or cholesteatoma.[6] Limitation of range of motion while opening the jaw is seen more often with conditions affecting the temporal muscles or temporal-mandibular join rather than deep infection. In many cases, advanced imaging is necessary to help rule out these listed conditions that are unrelated to the original ear surgery and to help locate the focus of infection for the purposes of surgical planning.[25]

INITIAL MANAGEMENT

Dogs presenting with suspicious clinical signs suggesting deep infection following TECA-LBO may be initially managed in a variety of ways. Depending on the financial concerns of the owner, it is not unreasonable to first determine if the patient's signs and quality of life improve with empirical antibiotic therapy and nonsteroidal antiinflammatory drugs (NSAIDs). Owners should understand that the improvement may be temporary, and further diagnostic imaging and surgery will be necessary should medical therapy fail or the condition recurs after antibiotics are discontinued. There are few reports documenting the long-term outcome following antibiotic therapy alone for recurrent deep infection; however, it seems that success is limited in many dogs.[11,12] Diagnostic imaging and surgery are expensive, and invasive surgery may be complicated and not necessarily successful on first attempt.[11] Therefore, it is sensible to initially consider an antibiotic trial in select cases.

Initial choice of antibiotics for treatment of deep infection may be based on culture and susceptibility results obtained from the original surgery. A variety of *Staphylococcal isolates*, *Escherichia coli*, *Enterococcus*, and beta-hemolytic *Streptococcus* were isolated in deep cultures following surgical exploration of fistulas and tympanic bulla in 1 report.[12] Similar bacterial isolates have been isolated within the tympanic bulla in other studies.[8,11,14,15] Keep in mind that more resistant bacteria (ie, *Pseudomonas aeruginosa* and *E coli*) are also commonly isolated from deep wound cultures in some reports.[8,14,26] Broad spectrum antibiotics, such as augmented penicillins or potentiated sulfonamides, may be good initial empirical antibiotic choices provided the patient has no known risks for adverse drug reactions.

First-generation cephalosporin antibiotics are not recommended because about only 25% of bacteria commonly isolated from the bulla during TECA-LBO are sensitive to this drug.[26]

Isolation of bacteria responsible for the deep focus of infection is a preferable method to help choose appropriate antibiotic therapy. When fistulation is present, do not attempt to obtain samples from the opening or discharge because superficial contaminants will confuse the susceptibility results. The author prefers to choose the appropriate antibiotic regimen based on deep culture results at the time of initial presentation. In the author' experience, ultrasound-guided fine-needle aspiration of deep fluid pockets has been a rewarding method to obtain samples for culture. The ideal antibiotic therapy duration has not been established; however, consider administration for at least 4 to 6 weeks, provided the patient shows a positive response and remains comfortable. The author has had some success keeping signs of infection in check by extending antibiotic therapy several months or longer when owners refuse further workup, or when other significant comorbidities take anesthesia and surgery out of consideration.

DIAGNOSTIC APPROACH

When surgical treatment is being considered, first determine if the dog is healthy enough to undergo anesthesia and rule out significant comorbidities. Advanced radiographic imaging is the next step in the diagnostic tree. The deep infection source should be accurately located, if possible, and other differential diagnoses (listed previously) should be ruled out before proceeding. Plain radiographic imaging may be helpful in identifying lesions affecting boney structures surrounding the tympanic bulla but it is not a consistently accurate tool to help identify the location of the infection focus.[25] However, the bulla as a focus of infection can be ruled out if it appears air-filled on oblique and open mouth views of the tympanic bulla. Lytic processes affecting regional boney structures suggest an underlying neoplastic process not discovered during the original surgery. In 1 study, increased opacity was consistently evident within the tympanic bulla when the infection was found to be located in this structure.[11] In this same study, no confirmed deep infections located within the bulla caused lysis or extensive boney proliferation. Sclerosis or ventrolateral flattening of the affected tympanic bulla, and increased soft tissue density within or just lateral to the osseous bulla, were evident in dogs that presented with facial fistulation caused by remnants of the horizontal ear canal after TECA-LBO.[12] In about 30% of these dogs, there was no specific plain radiographic lesion other than what is expected after a previous LBO.[12,24] Mcanulty and colleagues[24] found healing of the bulla after TECA-LBO in normal dogs was highly variable, and the bulla ostectomy site can either partially or completely reform, or the tympanic cavity can become filled with new bone. Plain films may identify a remnant of the horizontal ear canal when the ear canal cartilage is calcified because there should be no evidence of the horizontal ear canal left after a properly performed TECA-LBO.[13]

Contrast fistulograms may be considered in dogs with a single draining track but the contrast track may stop short of the deeper nidus. In 1 study, fistulograms performed in only 1 of 9 dogs showed contrast extending beyond the subcutaneous tissue plane. In these same dogs, the infection source was subsequently identified at surgery adjacent to the external auditory meatus.[12] In another study, contrast within the fistulous track extended to the ventrolateral tympanic bulla; however, it did not lead to the epithelial remnant within the tympanic cavity.[11] Therefore, fistulography may not be expected to reliably extend to the deep focus of infection.

CT imaging with contrast is the author's preferred diagnostic imaging modality for confirming the location of the deep infection. Contrast enhancement surrounds the source of the infection in most cases (**Fig. 2**).

Contrast CT imaging helps the surgeon determine which approach (lateral through the original incision site or ventral to the bulla) to best expose and remove the infection nidus without risking damage to important regional structures.

Because the tympanic cavity is best exposed through the ventral approach,[11,27] dissection is carried outside the original surgical site through virgin tissue and normal anatomic landmarks are preserved, it is the approach of choice for an infection focus isolated within the tympanic cavity.[11] The original surgical site is explored laterally when the nidus cannot be accurately located, or when the deep infection source is found to be adjacent and lateral to the external auditory meatus. This approach is also recommended when a horizontal canal remnant is identified because these structures are not readily exposed or removed via the ventral bulla approach.[12] MRI may be useful to evaluate invasive processes infiltrating deep structures, or when the patient shows neurologic signs suggestive of inner ear or multiple cranial nerve dysfunction, because these soft tissue structures are better identified with this modality.[28]

SURGICAL EXPLORATION

A lateral approach is always chosen when remnants of the horizontal canal and/or an infection nidus are identified by imaging lateral to the tympanic bulla (see **Fig. 2**). This

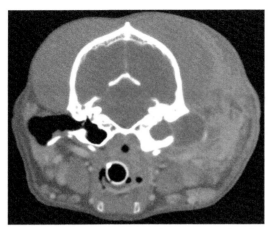

Fig. 2. Contrast CT image of a dog with a deep infection located within and just lateral to the incomplete left lateral bulla ostectomy during TECA. Note the irregular soft tissue densities (inflammatory tissue) lateral to the contrast-enhancing abscess. An air-filled right bulla and ear canal can be used for comparison.

approach will also allow access and more limited exposure of the tympanic cavity.[12] The disadvantage to this approach is that dissection is carried through dense scar and inflamed tissue, which makes identification of important landmarks and structures (facial nerve and large vessels) difficult and tedious. Consequently, the risk of facial nerve damage and profuse hemorrhage during surgery are concerns when exploration is conducted through this approach.[12]

Position the patient in lateral recumbency, with the affected side propped up with a cervical support such as a rolled towel. Aseptically prepare the entire region surrounding the ear and pinna, and extend the preparation to include any surrounding fistulous tracks. Create a vertical skin incision over the original TECA-LBO incision. If a fistula is present, and there is desire to explore and follow the track, extend the incision to include the track opening. With a combination of blunt and sharp dissection, explore the incision through the subcutaneous tissues toward the region of the external auditory meatus. This tissue is often very fibrotic and may require careful sharp dissection in the deeper aspects of the incision. If the external auditory meatus can be definitively located, bluntly tunnel a mosquito hemostatic forceps into the tympanic cavity. This serves as an important landmark to refer to during further dissection. If possible, it is best to isolate and preserve the facial nerve at this point in the dissection. Search for this delicate white linear structure caudal to the meatus exiting the stylomastoid foramen, and during dissection ventrolateral to the bulla. Avoid stray dissection, particularly in the region directly ventral to the auditory meatus and remaining tympanic bulla because this could damage important nearby vascular structures. Remnants of the horizontal ear canal generally appear as firm yellowish-white cartilage with a dark greenish-brown epithelial lining (**Fig. 3**). Remove all remnants of canal tissue from the opening of the external auditory meatus (osseous portion of the ear canal) with rongeurs. Dissect the soft tissue off the lateral face of the tympanic bulla with Freer periosteal elevators, and use rongeurs to remove enough of the remaining bulla to adequately expose the tympanic cavity.[13] Remove any greenish-brown epithelial remnants and debris from the external auditory meatus and tympanic cavity with curettes. Avoid curetting in the dorsal compartment and epitympanic recess of the tympanic cavity to reduce the risk of inner ear damage. This complication occurred

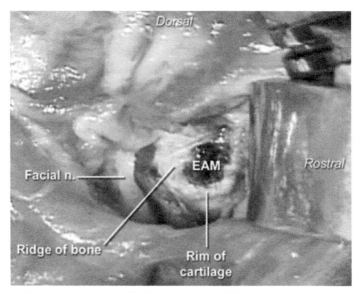

Fig. 3. Lateral approach to the bulla showing a rim of horizontal ear canal and greenish-brown epithelial lining. EAM, external auditory meatus; n., nerve.

in 2 out of 9 cases explored for fistula formation after TECA-LBO in 1 report.[12] Thoroughly irrigate the bulla to remove any remaining free bone pieces and debris. Take a sample of the debris and epithelium for culture and biopsy. There is no need to remove the ossicles if they are exposed. The author has found that the use of a sterile 30-degree 5 mm videoscope for final inspection of the entire tympanic cavity helps to identify any remaining debris and epithelium accidentally left in deep recesses.[29] Generally, the wound does not require drainage unless a substantial abscess is encountered during dissection. Thoroughly lavage the entire wound. Subcutaneous tissue and skin closure are routine. No bandaging is required.

A ventral bulla approach is indicated when there is no evidence of an infection focus lateral to the tympanic cavity, and CT imaging shows contrast enhancement deep within the tympanic cavity or external auditory meatus only[11,27] **(Fig. 4)**. This approach provides excellent exposure of the entire tympanic cavity, so it is the procedure of choice when the focus of infection is within this structure. However, realize that the ventral approach does not allow ready access to tissues lateral to the external auditory meatus. Dissection through virgin tissue planes is another advantage of this approach because the region ventral to the bulla is not generally affected by scar tissue from the original TECA-LBO approach. In contrast to the lateral approach, regional anatomic landmarks are preserved and the dissection plane should not cross the path of the facial nerve. The ventral bulla can be fully exposed so that important nearby vascular structures can be isolated and preserved.

Position the patient in dorsal recumbency with the neck extended over a cervical support. Aseptically prepare the skin from the midmandible to midventral cervical region. If possible, confirm the affected side and locate the dome-shaped bulla by deep digital palpation just caudomedial to the angular process of the mandible. Make a 7 to 10 cm rostrocaudal paramedian incision centered over the affected bulla. Continue sharp dissection through the platysma and sphincter colli muscles. Preserve the underlying linguofacial and maxillary veins. Bluntly separate the plane between the

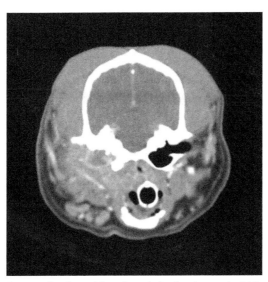

Fig. 4. Contrast CT image of a dog with a deep infection located within the previous right bulla ostectomy site. Notice the contrast enhancement surrounding the nidus of infection (epithelial remnant was found just inside the external auditory meatus).

digastricus and mylohyoid muscles. Bluntly dissect directly over the bulla through the hyoglossus and styloglossus muscles, and keep this tissue plane widely separated with Gelpi retractors to expose the entire ventral aspect of the tympanic bulla. Do not damage the hypoglossal nerve (medial side) and facial nerve (lateral side) by the sharp retractor tips. Isolate surrounding vascular structures, and sharply incise and dissect periosteum off the bulla with Freer periosteal elevators. If necessary, use a pin or powered burr to penetrate the central aspect of the ventral bulla. Enlarge the hole carefully with rongeurs or burr so the entire bulla cavity can be inspected. Just lateral to the tympanic bulla, the author routinely removes the ventral portion of the external auditory meatus to search for epithelium or remnants of the tympanum remaining in this region.

Avoid damaging inner ear structures in the promontory area when the bulla is first penetrated by a pin or burr, and during curettage of the bulla cavity. Use small curettes and hemostats to gently probe and remove debris and epithelial remnants. Epithelium generally appears as dark greenish-brown tissue (**Fig. 5**). Expect these remnants to be firmly adhered to the underlying bone so forceful curettage may be necessary. Remember to carefully scrape or gently pull away abnormal tissue from the sensitive inner ear structures housed in the dorsal promontory region. Submit epithelial or debris samples for culture and biopsy. If remnants of the tympanum are found just within the epitympanic recess, the stapes is removed with the remnant; however, there is no need to remove the incus and malleus if they are exposed. Irrigate the tympanic cavity thoroughly before separate closure of the muscle, subcutaneous layer, and skin. Wound drainage and bandaging are generally not indicated.

POSTOPERATIVE MONITORING AND CARE

Deep exploration of the region lateral to the external auditory meatus and ventral to the bulla can be challenging and result in early postoperative hemorrhage, pharyngeal

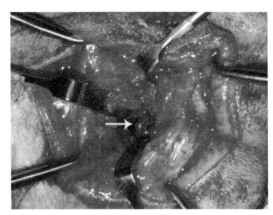

Fig. 5. Ventral exploration of the bulla TECA-LBO surgery. A discolored epithelial remnant is visible (*white arrow*) in the middle of the image.

swelling, upper respiratory obstruction, and extreme pain. Ventilation should be monitored diligently and direct arterial blood pressure monitoring should be considered until the patient is fully recovered from anesthesia. Dogs are usually given continuous infusions of opioids, such as fentanyl, often with the addition of ketamine and lidocaine to provide a comfortable postoperative recovery. If not contraindicated, the addition of an NSAID, such as carprofen, is helpful in reducing the inflammation from aggressive tissue dissection. Continuous wound infusion of local anesthetics may be helpful in controlling pain without the sedation and drug side effects associated with high doses of narcotics.[30] Pain can usually be controlled with an NSAID and tramadol, generally by 24 hours following surgery. Monitor and treat any ocular complications, especially corneal ulcers, if the patient is exophthalmic, or if there is evidence of keratoconjunctivitis sicca or facial nerve deficits. Acute surgical site infection should be treated with antibiotics and open wound drainage. The choice of antibiotic therapy after surgery should be based on the intraoperative culture and susceptibility results. The appropriate duration of antibiotic administration after surgery has not been determined but the author recommends at least 2 weeks.

Owners should be educated about clinical signs suggesting recurrence of infection. Swelling noted lateral or ventral to the incision, pain elicited on palpation of the incision area, or when opening the jaw should prompt the owner to seek veterinary care.

OUTCOME
Antibiotic Therapy Alone

It seems that clinical signs from deep infection following TECA-LBO can often be held in check with antibiotics but recurrence after antibiotic withdrawal is common.[11,12] Of the 3 dogs that were treated with intermittent empirical antibiotic therapy for recurrent fistula formation in Holt's study, 1 dog had no recurrence after 1 course of antibiotics for a follow-up of 12 months, and 2 dogs had only temporary resolution of signs when antibiotics were administered.[12] Infection resolved after 5 years of intermittent antibiotic treatment in 1 dog, and in the other dog, signs of deep infection eventually resolved following several of courses of antibiotics after 12 months. In Matthieson's study, antibiotic therapy was initially successful at eliminating clinical signs in the only dog developing deep infection following TECA-LBO.[17] Signs recurred and antibiotic therapy was reinstituted, and the dog had no further signs for a follow-up of

12 months. Antibiotic therapy was successful in permanently resolving deep infection in only 1 of 9 dogs in Smeak's report.[11] The remaining dogs initially treated with antibiotics responded for several weeks, but signs recurred and the dogs eventually underwent surgical treatment. Provided clinical signs improve and the pet is comfortable, intermittent antibiotic therapy can be offered, especially when owners are not interested in more aggressive surgical therapy. Some dogs will ultimately have resolution of clinical signs of deep infection after prolonged (months to years) antibiotic therapy.

Surgical Therapy

Surgical exploration offers the most consistently successful therapy for treatment of deep infection, but the outcome is not always positive. In Holt and colleagues[12] study, after failed antibiotic attempts, 7 of 10 dogs had permanent resolution of fistula formation following TECA-LBO when explored through a lateral approach. Deep infection was resolved in all 3 dogs that were explored via the ventral approach in Mason and colleagues[18] study. The only dog developing deep infection in another case series had resolution after bulla exploration through a ventral approach.[20] Three of 4 dogs explored for deep infection through a ventral approach were successful in an early retrospective study of dogs undergoing TECA.[15] However, in a later study by the same investigator, only 1 of 7 dogs explored for deep infection from a ventral approach had permanent resolution of clinical signs on the first exploratory attempt.[11] However, of the 5 dogs with recurrence of infection following exploration that were surgically re-explored through the same approach, all had permanent resolution of the infection. Of the 2 dogs that developed deep infection in another report, surgery was successful in 1 dog when explored through a lateral approach to remove a remnant of the horizontal canal. The other dog, explored initially via a ventral approach, that was re-explored through a lateral approach did not respond long-term and was eventually euthanatized.[19] This suggests that surgeons contemplating deep wound exploration should carefully plan the best approach to help thoroughly explore the wound to avoid missing an infected nidus deep within the original wound or bulla.

When dogs require exploratory surgery for recurrence of infection, postoperative complications are common, especially when a lateral approach is used. Neurologic complications, such as head tilt, otitis interna, and facial nerve paralysis, have been reported.[11,12] Facial nerve paralysis and otitis interna occurred after lateral exploration of fistulas in 2 out of 10 dogs.[12] Most neurologic complications will improve over time but owners should be advised that some remain permanent.[12] Because the stakes are high, and owners generally consider exploration a last-ditch effort, surgeons likely are more aggressive with their dissection to thoroughly expose the deep wound, and during curettage of the bulla, to ensure complete removal of epithelium and debris in the bulla. Firm scar tissue and abnormal or absent tissue planes encountered during surgical exploration obscure anatomic landmarks, and this can lead to stray dissection and damage to deep neurovascular structures.

SUMMARY

Surgeons must attempt to carefully remove all of the ear canal and epithelium within the external auditory meatus and tympanic cavity to help avoid deep infection complications following TECA-LBO. When persistent deep infection or fistulation forms after ablation, clinical signs can be more debilitating than the initial signs related to the otitis externa or media. Clinical signs of deep infection can be relieved with appropriate antibiotic therapy but recurrence is common. Prolonged courses of antibiotics can be successful in permanent resolution of deep infection in a minority of affected dogs. When the clinical signs of deep infection are not relieved with antibiotic therapy, or become recalcitrant, surgical exploration is recommended. Contrast CT imaging is particularly helpful in locating the nidus of infection. A lateral approach through the original incision is suggested if the nidus of infection cannot be conclusively identified with advanced imaging because the entire original wound can be explored along with the osseous ear canal and tympanic cavity. However, exposure is often limited through the lateral approach and neurologic complications after re-exploration are not uncommon. If the nidus is definitively isolated within the bulla or external auditory meatus, a ventral approach is preferred because deeper dissection is not constrained by scar tissue and wide exposure can be achieved. In addition, the facial nerve can be easily preserved because it lies lateral to the ventral approach plane. Surgery is often ultimately successful in resolving deep infection if performed carefully by an experienced surgeon. Surgical re-exploration or, alternately, long-term antibiotic therapy can be successful in alleviating clinical signs of infection when deep infection occurs after exploration.

REFERENCES

1. Smeak DD, Kerpsack SJ. Total ear canal ablation and lateral bulla osteotomy for management of end-stage otitis. Semin Vet Med Surg (Small Anim) 1993;8(1): 30–41.
2. Devitt CM, Seim HB 3rd, Willer R, et al. Passive drainage versus primary closure after total ear canal ablation-lateral bulla osteotomy in dogs: 59 dogs (1985-1995). Vet Surg 1997;26(3):210–6.
3. Angus JC, Lichtensteiger C, Campbell KL, et al. Breed variations in histopathologic features of chronic severe otitis external in dogs: 80 cases (1995-2001). J Am Vet Med Assoc 2002;221(7):1000–6.
4. Moltzen H. Canine ear disease. J Small Anim Pract 1969;10:589–92.
5. Little CJ, Lane JG, Person GR. Inflammatory middle ear disease of the dog: the pathology of otitis media. Vet Rec 1991;128:293–6.
6. Hardie EM, Linder KE, Pease AP. Aural cholesteatoma in twenty dogs. Vet Surg 2008;37(8):763–70.
7. White RAS, Pomeroy CJ. Total ear canal ablation and lateral bulla osteotomy in the dog. J Small Anim Pract 1990;31(11):547–53.
8. Spivack RE, Elkins AD, Moore GE, et al. Postoperative complications following TECA-LBO in the dog and cat. J Am Anim Hosp Assoc 2013;49(3):160–8.
9. Cole LK, Kwochka KW, Hillier A, et al. Comparison of bacterial organisms and their susceptibility patterns from otic exudate and ear tissue from the vertical ear canal of dogs undergoing total ear canal ablation. Vet Ther 2005;6(3):252–9.
10. Smeak DD. Total ear canal ablation and lateral bulla osteotomy. In: Monnet E, editor. Small animal soft tissue surgery, vol. 1, 1st edition. Ames (IA): Wiley-Blackwell; 2013. p. 132–44.
11. Smeak DD, Crocker CB, Birchard SJ. Treatment of recurrent otitis media that developed after total ear canal ablation and lateral bulla osteotomy in dogs: nine cases (1986-1994). J Am Vet Med Assoc 1996;209(5):937–42.
12. Holt D, Brockman DJ, Sylvestre AM, et al. Lateral exploration of fistulas developing after total ear canal ablations: 10 cases (1989-1993). J Am Anim Hosp Assoc 1996;32(6):527–30.

13. Smeak DD, Inpanbutr N. Lateral approach to subtotal bulla osteotomy in dogs: pertinent anatomy and procedural details. Comp Cont Educ Prac Vet 2005;27: 377–84.

14. Hettlich BE, Boothe HW, Simpson RB, et al. Effect of tympanic cavity evacuation and flushing on microbial isolates during total ear canal ablation with lateral bulla osteotomy in dogs. J Am Vet Med Assoc 2005;227(5):748–55.

15. Smeak DD, Dehoff WD. Total ear canal ablation: clinical results in the dog and cat. Vet Surg 1986;15(2):161–70.

16. Smeak DD. Management of complications associated with total ear canal ablation and bulla osteotomy in dogs and cats. Vet Clin North Am Small Anim Pract 2011;41(5):981–94.

17. Matthiesen DT, Scavelli T. Total ear canal ablation and lateral bulla osteotomy in 38 dogs. J Am Anim Hosp Assoc 1990;26(3):257–67.

18. Mason LK, Harvey CE, Orsher RJ. Total ear canal ablation combined with lateral bulla osteotomy for end-stage otitis in dogs - results in 30 dogs. Vet Surg 1988; 17(5):263–8.

19. Sharp NJ. Chronic otitis-externa and otitis-media treated by total ear canal ablation and ventral bulla osteotomy in 13 dogs. Vet Surg 1990;19(2):162–6.

20. Beckman SL, Henry WB Jr, Cechner P. Total ear canal ablation combining bulla osteotomy and curettage in dogs with chronic otitis externa and media. J Am Vet Med Assoc 1990;196(1):84–90.

21. Williams JM, White RAS. Total ear canal ablation combined with lateral bulla osteotomy in the cat. J Small Anim Pract 1992;33(5):225–7.

22. Bacon NJ, Gilbert RL, Bostock DE, et al. Total ear canal ablation in the cat: indications, morbidity and long-term survival. J Small Anim Pract 2003;44(10):430–4.

23. Marino DJ, MacDonald JM, Matthieson DT, et al. Results of surgery in cats with ceruminous gland adenocarcinoma. J Am Anim Hosp Assoc 1994;30:54–8.

24. Mcanulty JF, Hattel A, Harvey CE. Wound-healing and brain-stem auditory-evoked potentials after experimental total ear canal ablation with lateral tympanic bulla osteotomy in dogs. Vet Surg 1995;24(1):1–8.

25. Garosi LS, Dennis R, Schwarz T. Review of diagnostic imaging of ear diseases in the dog and cat. Vet Radiol Ultrasound 2003;44(2):137–46.

26. Vogel PL, Komtebedde J, Hirsh DC, et al. Wound contamination and antimicrobial susceptibility of bacteria cultured during total ear canal ablation and lateral bulla osteotomy in dogs. J Am Vet Med Assoc 1999;214(11):1641–3.

27. Mcanulty JF, Harvey CE, Hattel A. A preliminary-study of the effects of ventral bulla osteotomy and total ear canal ablation with lateral bulla osteotomy. Vet Surg 1985;14(1):60.

28. Harran XH, Bradley KJ, Hetzel N, et al. MRI findings of a middle ear cholesteatoma in a dog. J Am Anim Hosp Assoc 2012;48:185–9.

29. Haudiquet PH, Gauthier O, Renard E. Total ear canal ablation associated with lateral bulla ostectomy with the help of otoscopy in dogs and cats: retrospective study of 47 cases. Vet Surg 2006;35(4):E1–20.

30. Wolfe TM, Bateman SW, Cole LK, et al. Evaluation of a local anesthetic delivery system for the postoperative analgesic management of canine total ear canal ablation - a randomized, controlled, double-blinded study. Vet Anaesth Analg 2006;33(5):328–39.

Diagnosis and Management of Cholesteatomas in Dogs

Marije Risselada, DVM, PhD

KEYWORDS

- Cholesteatoma • Middle ear • Diagnosis • Imaging • Surgical management

KEY POINTS

- Aural cholesteatomas are expansile lesions of the middle ear.
- Clinical symptoms are draining tracts, pain on opening the mouth, and neurologic impairment.
- Imaging findings include soft tissue density in the middle ear and destruction of the bone of the bulla with characteristics of an aggressive lesion.
- Patients with neurologic signs have a poorer prognosis.
- Long-term medical treatment of recurring or persisting signs is possible.

INTRODUCTION

Nature of the Problem

A middle ear cholesteatoma is an expansile lesion of the middle ear; it presents as a lesion that can be locally destructive, giving the appearance of an aggressive tumor, although it is a non-neoplastic condition.

This lesion consists of an epidermoid cyst that contains keratin debris and is lined by keratinizing squamous epithelium.[1–6] The keratotic material is accumulated because of secondary hyperkeratosis from misplaced keratinizing stratified squamous epithelium within the lesion. This accumulation leads to gradual enlargement of the cyst causing compression and potentially destruction of the surrounding tissues.[5] Expansion and rupture of the cyst cause an inflammatory condition and can become infected, as evidenced by positive cultures in most cases. This secondary infection of the cyst will then increase the inflammatory reaction exacerbating the response.[1]

In veterinary patients, this condition was initially thought to be secondary to a failed total ear canal ablation-lateral bulla osteotomy (TECA-LBO) procedure for otitis externa and media but has been proven to develop as a primary condition or

The author has nothing to disclose.
Department of Clinical Sciences, College of Veterinary Medicine, North Carolina State University, Veterinary Health Complex, 1052 William Moore Drive, Raleigh, NC 27607, USA
E-mail address: marije_risselada@ncsu.edu

Vet Clin Small Anim 46 (2016) 623–634
http://dx.doi.org/10.1016/j.cvsm.2016.01.002
0195-5616/16/$ – see front matter Published by Elsevier Inc.

component of otitis externa/media without prior surgery or iatrogenic trauma, as shown in a large case series.[1] The incidence of cholesteatoma in dogs with otitis media could be as high as 11%.[7]

Although the etiopathogenesis is not completely understood, by consensus, 2 broad categories are currently recognized: congenital and acquired (**Table 1**).[6] The congenital form is rare and has not been reported in dogs.[1–4] It is defined as a expanding cystic mass assumed to be present at birth but usually diagnosed in infancy or early childhood.[6]

The development of the congenital form can be further subclassified in the epithelial rest theory and the acquired inclusion theory.[5] In the epithelial rest theory, it is proposed that a nest of epithelial cells pathologically persist in the fetal temporal bones. If the cells are implanted into the middle ear because of a childhood event affecting the tympanic membrane (TM) or middle ear, it is termed *acquired inclusion*.[5]

Acquired cholesteatomas can be categorized according to their proposed pathogenesis into 4 different categories: a primary form and 3 secondary forms.[1–4] The primary form is thought to develop secondary to a dysfunction of the eustachian tube and chronic misventilation of the auditory tube, which in turn leads to invagination of the TM into the bulla (invagination or retraction theory).[2,4] Ligation of the eustachian tube in gerbils did induce cholesteatomas in 75% of animals in one study, but experimental ligation of the eustachian tube in other studies did not induce cholesteatomas.[8]

The secondary form is considered secondary to chronic otitis media, trauma to the middle ear, or secondary to surgery of the external ear canal and middle ear.[1–4] The metaplasia theory posits that the normally present modified ciliated respiratory epithelium in the bulla undergoes a metaplastic transformation into stratified squamous epithelium because of chronic inflammation. A second theory suggests that breaks in the TM (perforations, rupture, or after surgery) can lead to migration of the stratified squamous epithelium from the external ear canal into the tympanic bulla where it can lead to keratin formation and accumulation due to chronic inflammation (migration theory). The third theory (invasion theory) proposes that keratinizing epithelial cells of the TM migrate into the subepithelial space of the bulla through a basement membrane breach.

Regardless of the cause, the cholesteatoma expands and gradually erodes neighboring bone structures, after which it can expand further,[9] potentially explaining the lytic nature of the bone of the affected tympanic bulla. It has been hypothesized that osteoclasts might be activated during the formation of cholesteatomas and implicated in the bony lysis of the bulla. Osteoclasts have been found microscopically, leading to theorize about their possible involvement.[10–12] However, activated osteoclasts were not identified in bone collected from dogs with cholesteatomatous otitis media in a recent case series.[9]

Definition
It is an expansile cyst containing keratotic material in the middle ear.

Symptom Criteria

- Expansile lesion in the bulla
- Chronic otitis externa/media
- Presence or absence of pain on opening of the jaw
- Presence or absence of neurologic signs, either due to destruction of the petrous bone or due to facial nerve palsy

Table 1
Classification and etiopathogenesis of middle ear cholesteatomas

	Acquired		Congenital (Rare)
	Primary	Secondary	
Cause	Chronic misventilation of the auditory tube	Complication of otitis media or trauma	Dispersed cells during embryogenesis
Pathogenesis	The TM retracts into the TC leading to adhesions and cholesteatoma formation	Metaplasia of the epithelium into stratified squamous epithelium due to chronic inflammation	Migration of squamous epithelium into the TC after a trigger (inflammatory process) and across a bridge (granulation tissue) through perforations in or rupture of the TM	Invasion of epithelial cells into subepithelial space through a BM breach	No inflammatory trigger or defects are needed
Synonyms	Invagination theory Retraction theory	Metaplasia theory	Migration theory	Invasion theory	—
Species	Humans	Humans, dogs			Humans, Mongolian gerbil

Abbreviations: BM, basement membrane; TC, tympanic chamber; TM, tympanic membrane.
Data from Refs.[1–4]

CLINICAL FINDINGS
Signalment and History

No significant breed predilection has been reported in the literature, although spaniels and retrievers seem to be overrepresented (pugs [3], spaniels [10], and retrievers [6]),[1,3,4,13] and a higher incidence in male dogs was found; but this finding was not significant, most likely because of small patient numbers. In people, a similar, as of yet unexplained, sex bias has been reported.[14]

Although cholesteatomas are most commonly found in middle-aged to older dogs, the reported ages on presentation in the literature range from 2 to 12 years old.[1,3] Similarly, most dogs present with a protracted history of aural disease, although the reported duration of signs is variable, ranging from 3 weeks to more than 6 years.[1,3]

Presenting complaints include otitis externa, head shaking, pain on opening of the mouth or inability to fully open the mouth, and neurologic signs.[1,3,4,13]

Most cases reported in the veterinary literature have unilateral disease. In the earlier large case series by Hardie and colleagues,[1] 15 out of 19 patients had unilateral disease. In subsequent more recent articles, all but one case were unilateral (**Table 2**).[1,3,4,13]

The incidence of prior surgery varied extensively between the different studies: Hardie and colleagues[1] reported that 3 of the 20 included patients had had prior surgery (TECA-LBO 1, lateral wall resection 1, external ear canal mass resection 1), whereas all included cases in 2 other studies underwent surgery before presentation: The 2 patients reported by Schuenemann and Oechtering[4] had an LBO performed previously; and of the 11 patients reported by Greci and colleagues,[3] 10 underwent a TECA-LBO previously and one a VBO.

Physical Examination

Presenting complaints include signs related to chronic otitis externa/media (head shaking, pain on palpation, discharge, swelling, redness, ±draining tracts), pain on opening of the mouth or inability to fully open the mouth, and neurologic signs, including head tilt, facial nerve palsy, ataxia, and nystagmus.

Inability to open the mouth or discomfort on opening of the mouth is a common presenting complaint, reported in 6 out of 10 dogs[3] and 4 out of 20 dogs.[1] Respiratory signs can be present due to a space-occupying mass compromising the lumen of the nasopharynx/larynx, as reported by Schuenemann and Oechtering.[4]

Otoscopic Examination

Most dogs showed pain on palpation of the area of the bulla (9 out of 10 dogs) and/or otorrhea (8 out of 10 dogs).[3] Findings during an otoscopic or video otoscopic examination can resemble end-stage otitis externa. Greci and colleagues[3] described a total occlusion of the horizontal canal in 4 out of 11 ears with end-stage otitis. In other cases the external ear canal can be patent, allowing visualization of the cholesteatoma itself. These cholesteatomas appear as a pearly white to yellow growth protruding from the middle ear cavity into the external ear canal (Newman and colleagues,[5] 2015, one case) (Greci and colleagues,[3] 2011, 3 cases).

Focused Neurologic Examination

More than 50% of dogs present with concurrent neurologic signs, or neurologic abnormalities were found on physical examination (head tilt, facial nerve paralysis, ataxia) in 5 out of 10 dogs[3] and 7 out of 20 dogs.[1] The presence or absence of neurologic signs can serve as a prognostic indicator for recurrence of symptoms or disease after surgical treatment.[1]

Table 2
Imaging findings described in the veterinary literature

	Radiographs (1 out of 1)[3]	CT	MR (1 out of 1)[13]
Unilateral vs bilateral	Unilateral	Unilateral (15 out of 19)[1] (11 out of 11)[2] (10 out of 11)[3]	—
Middle ear contents	Loss of air contrast	Soft tissue density or soft tissue–like material	Isointense to brain tissue (T1W) Mixed intensity (T2W & FLAIR)
Bulla	Sclerosis of the tympanic wall Expansion of the bulla	Osteoproliferation (13 out of 19)[1] (9 out of 11)[2] (9 out of 11)[3] Lysis of the bulla (12 out of 19)[1] (8 out of 11)[2] (5 out of 11)[3] Expansion of the bulla (11 out of 19)[1] (10 out of 11)[2] (11 out of 11)[3]	Expanded bulla Thickened and irregularly shaped wall: hypointense (T1W), mixed intensity (T2W)
Calvarium	Sclerosis of petrosal bone	Bone lysis within the squamous or petrosal portions of the temporal bone (4 out of 19)[1] (5 out of 11)[2]	Petrous temporal bone hypointense on T1W and T2W images
Soft tissue	—	Lymph node enlargement (7 out of 19)[1]	—
TMJ	—	Sclerosis of ipsilateral TMJ (10 out of 11)[2,3]	—
Contrast	—	Contrast enhancement of the tissue in the middle ear (7 out of 10)[1] No contrast enhancement of the tissue in the middle ear (11 out of 11)[2,3] Peripheral ring enhancement (4 out of 11)[2]	Partial enhancement of inner lining (T1W)

Abbreviations: CT, computed tomography; FLAIR, fluid-attenuated inversion recovery; MR, magnetic resonance; T1W, T1 weighted; T2W, T2 weighted; TMJ, temporomandibular joint.
Data from Refs.[1–3,13]

IMAGING

Although different modalities are discussed, computed tomography (CT) or alternatively magnetic resonance (MR) are the methods of choice for assessing the middle ear and middle-ear associated lesions, as they provide improved detail for lesions in areas of complex architecture (see **Table 2**).[15]

Radiographs

A radiographic evaluation might be chosen as a first-line assessment or in the absence of access to either CT or MR. It should ideally be performed under anesthesia and should include a lateral view, a 20° lateral oblique view, a dorsoventral view, and a rostrocaudal open mouth view to best visualize the individual bullae. Described radiographic features of chronic otitis media include lack of air in the bulla, thickening of the bulla wall, and with or without increased size of the bulla; however, the external ear canal can be air filled. Radiographic features of neoplasia include lysis of the bulla and bony proliferation with or without soft tissue lesion filling or extending into the bulla. These findings are nonspecific and can be found in otitis media as well as other lesions affecting the tympanic bulla.[15]

Ultrasonography

The use of ultrasonography has been described in assessing middle ear lesions but has been determined to be less accurate than radiographs and highly operator dependent.[16] It might, however, be of value for obtaining either fine-needle aspiration or true-cut biopsy samples.

Computed Tomography

Reported findings of the tympanic bulla include osteoproliferation, lysis, and sclerosis. The bulla is expanded (**Figs. 1–3**) and filled with soft tissue–like material. The external ear canal can be involved and filled with fluid or soft tissue, although in other cases the external ear canal can be air filled (see **Fig. 2**).

Bone lysis within the squamous or petrosal portions of the temporal bone have been described in 25% (Hardie and colleagues[1]) to 50% (Greci and colleagues[3]) of cases.

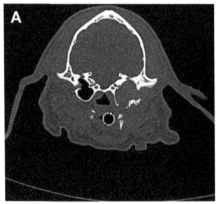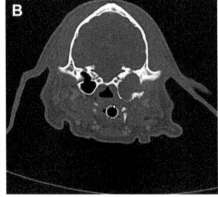

Fig. 1. A transverse image of a CT of a 7-year-old male castrated cocker spaniel with a left-sided cholesteatoma. (*A*) Before contrast and (*B*) after contrast administration. An expansile soft tissue mass of the left tympanic bulla is shown with sclerosis of the left temporal bone. The wall of the bulla shows lytic areas as well as thickening and remodeling. The mass itself is minimally contrast enhancing.

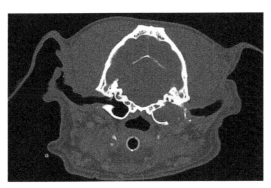

Fig. 2. A transverse image of a CT of a 6-year-old male castrated mixed breed dog with a left-sided cholesteatoma. Note the noninvolvement of the external ear canal and the expansion and destruction of the bulla. A soft tissue attenuating mass expands and fills the entire left tympanic bulla. The ventral margin of the bulla is thin and disrupted; the lesion is localized to the middle ear cavity.

Initial reports indicated that the tissue in the bulla enhances after contrast administration; however, later descriptions further define the contrast enhancement to be only localized around the lining of the bulla and not to involve the entire soft tissue structure filling the bulla.[3] Other reports indicate that contrast enhancement of the epithelial lining of the tympanic bulla in chronic otitis media cases is confined to an area directly adjacent to the bone (Garosi and colleagues[15]), similar to cholesteatomas. Neoplastic lesions are most commonly an extension of external ear canal tumors into the bulla, and contrast enhancement of the mass within the external ear canal might allow differentiation. Aggressive neoplastic lesions originating within the tympanic bulla are extremely rare but might exhibit some of the same features, such as filling of the bulla with soft tissue and lysis of the bulla wall, but do not typically exhibit the same general expansion of the entire tympanic bulla.

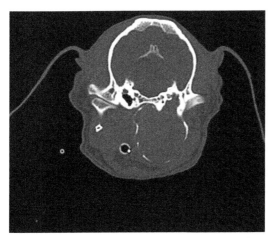

Fig. 3. A noncontrast transverse image of a CT of a 10-year-old male castrated shih tzu is shown with a left-sided cholesteatoma. The left tympanic bulla is severely expanded and is filled with a soft tissue mass. The expanded bulla attenuates the nasopharynx and is markedly attenuating and displacing the oropharynx and larynx to the right. The temporal and masseter muscles on the left are atrophied compared with the contralateral side.

Other findings include enlargement of the local lymph nodes (7 out 19 cases)[1] or sclerosis of the ipsilateral temporomandibular joint in 10 of 11 patients.[3]

MRI

MR has been used to further define the intracranial extent of the disease or in the absence of CT imaging capabilities on site.[1,5,13,17] MR is better suited to define the soft tissue structures, such as nerves, vessels, and inner ear structures, whereas CT is better suited to assess the bony structures.[15]

MR findings include a severely expanded bulla containing material isointense to brain tissue on T1-weighted and of mixed intensity on T2-weighted and fluid-attenuated inversion recovery (FLAIR) images.[13] Similar to the CT findings, the tissue in the tympanic bulla was found to be minimally contrast enhancing, with contrast enhancement localized to the area immediately adjacent to the bone, in the location of the inner (epithelial) lining of the bulla.[5] Other findings include lysis of the petrous temporal bone.[5] MR features of neoplasia of the tympanic bulla have been described, but the number of cases in the literature might be too low to define distinct characteristics between cholesteatomas of the middle ear and malignant neoplasia of the middle ear.

Differential Diagnoses

Differential diagnoses to be considered are chronic otitis externa/media and aural neoplasia, either extending from the external canal into the tympanic bulla or neoplasia arising from the bulla.

In chronic otitis media, CT would also show a bulla filled with tissue or fluid, with or without lysis of the bone of the bulla, but lacks the expansile nature of growth and expansion of the bulla.

Neoplasia of the tympanic bulla in dogs is very rare. The most commonly described neoplasias extend from the external ear canal into the bulla (such as ceruminous gland adenoma, ceruminous gland adenocarcinoma, squamous cell carcinoma).[18] Contrast enhancement of the external portion of the mass could help differentiate between these and middle ear cholesteatomas and middle ear neoplasia.

Imaging findings that are described for middle ear neoplasia are similar to imaging findings for middle ear cholesteatomas but seem to have more contrast enhancement than cholesteatomas. Histologic sampling would be the only definitive differentiation between cholesteatomas and neoplastic lesions; but the otoscopic, cytologic, and imaging findings, in addition to the very rare incidence of primary middle ear neoplasia, should make middle ear cholesteatoma the primary differential.

PATHOLOGY
Cytology

Impression smears taken of a biopsy in one report revealed anucleate squamous epithelial cells, low numbers of inflammatory cells, small groups of spindle cells (presumed fibroblasts), and extracellular bacteria (cocci).[5]

Histopathology

Biopsy results are consistent with finding keratinizing epithelium and keratin debris (6 ears).[3]

A core of fibrous connective tissue can be present, covered by a hyperplastic keratinizing stratified squamous epithelium. A cystic lesion lined by a multilayered intensely hyperplastic keratinizing epithelium has also been described.[3]

In the submucosal layer, a large accumulation of cholesterol clefts was present, whereas the center of the lesion contained areas of mineralization and fragments of woven bone, leading to the histopathologic diagnosis of a cholesterol granuloma with osseous metaplasia (incisional biopsy).[5]

Microbiology

The culture results reflect a similar outcome as would be expected in chronic otitis externa cases. Hardie and colleagues[1] found positive aerobic cultures in 14 out of 16 cultured ears, with 3 dogs having more than 1 bacterial species cultured. Greci and colleagues[3] reported positive aerobic cultures from 8 out of 12 ears, and more than one species was recovered from one ear. *Staphylococcus* species were the most prevalent, with *Enterococcus* spp, *Pseudomonas aeruginosa*, *Staphylococcus* spp (3), *Proteus* (2), *Pseudomonas*, and *Escherichia coli* (1) making up the remainder of reported bacteria.[1,3]

A recent retrospective study on patients with chronic otitis externa/media reported positive cultures in 89% of cultured ears (n = 127), with *Staphylococcus* spp in 43% of ears, and found *Enterococcus* spp, *Pseudomonas*, *E coli*, and *Proteus mirabilis*.[18]

TREATMENT
Surgery

Surgical treatment can be curative in 50% of cases. Early surgical intervention is preferred; but even in later stage disease, surgery is recommended to remove the diseased tissue and remove as much of the space-occupying soft tissue and lesion, both from a diagnostic and from a palliative approach. Palliation might be obtained by removing the painful stimulus by removing the material from the bulla.

A caudal auricular approach has been described, but a ventral or lateral approach to the bulla is favored for the initial surgical treatment. The caudal approach was described in an attempt to preserve hearing and cosmetic outcome by preserving the external ear canal and reconstructing the ossicles.[19] A ventral approach has been preferentially used for cases with recurrent disease, especially if a lateral approach has been used previously, as it will provide better exposure to the bulla.[1,3,19]

Cases with chronic otitis externa are treated by TECA-LBO, as the disease involves both the external ear canal and the bulla (see **Fig. 1**). In these cases, the middle ear cholesteatoma could be an extension of the chronic disease in the external ear, with destruction of the tympanic membrane, allowing ingrowth of metaplastic ear canal epithelium into the middle ear. Care is taken to create good access to the tympanic cavity allowing for aggressive removal of the diseased tissue. If the expansive lesion of the bulla cannot be adequately accessed through a lateral approach, a combination of a lateral and ventral approach can be used to maximize exposure.[3] Complete removal is the goal of curative-intent surgery, and inspection of the bulla to check for remaining diseased tissue can be performed with an endoscope to facilitate this. Additionally, care must be taken not to transplant stratified squamous epithelium from the external ear canal into the middle ear during surgery, as this is one of proposed etiopathogeneses of canine middle ear cholesteatomas.[1]

In some cases the cholesteatoma of the middle ear can be contained within the middle ear, without overt external ear canal involvement (see **Fig. 2**). In such cases, a ventral approach (ventral bulla osteotomy [VBO]) can be used. Care must be taken to ensure that there is no diseased tissue in the external meatus. Magnification, such as surgical loupes, could help guide surgical dissection and removal of the tissue.

Regardless of the approach used, care is taken to remove as much of the diseased tissue as possible. Microscopic or endoscopic visualization, or a combination of both, is used in the surgical management of people with middle ear cholesteatomas.[20] This visualization might also help identify neurovascular structures more readily.

No difference in outcome was found between cases managed by a lateral approach or ventral approach. Cases managed with a TECA-LBO, or LBO only if a TECA had been performed previously, were evenly distributed over the 2 groups in the article by Hardie and colleagues.[1] They found that the cured cases had a lateral approach in 5 and a ventral approach in 4 cases, whereas the cases with recurrence had a lateral approach in 8 and a ventral in 2 patients. Three cases that had a second surgery all had a lateral approach in the revision surgery.[1]

It is key to remove all diseased/affected tissue to prevent recurrence. However, even in cases whereby removal was incomplete because of proximity of vital structures, a long-term survival was achieved despite needing chronic intermittent broad-spectrum antibiotics.[1,3]

Postoperative complications include facial nerve palsy/paresis/paralysis, recurrence of signs, development of draining tracts, and failure to resolve the preexisting neurologic signs.[1] These numbers are similar to the reported postoperative complication rates for TECA-LBO in dogs for otitis externa/interna[18] or VBO in dogs.

Medical Management

Chronic antibiotic therapy has been described for management in cases with recurrence after surgery or in cases whereby surgery was declined. The disease unfortunately is progressive, and the continued expansion of the cholesteatoma will lead to worsening of neurologic and/or respiratory signs over time.

PROGNOSIS/RECURRENCE

The combined reported rate of ears without recurrence after surgical therapy is 50%. In the case series by Hardie and colleagues,[1] 9 dogs had no recurrence and 10 had persistent or recurrent signs, whereas in the case series by Greci and colleagues,[3] 7 ears had no recurrence.

Greci and colleagues[3] reported a mean time until recurrence of 7.5 months (range 2–13 months postoperatively, 5 ears, confirmed in 4). Of the noncured animals in the study by Hardie and colleagues,[1] 5 dogs were readmitted for neurologic signs 1 to 16 months postoperatively. Three dogs were readmitted for inability to open the mouth at 2, 16, and 31 months postoperatively and underwent a second surgery (lateral approach) and, although requiring chronic intermittent antibiotic therapy, did not die of their cholesteatoma (37, 40, >52 months after the first surgery).

Clinical signs on presentation or imaging that were found to have a significant effect on the development of recurrence (univariate analysis) were inability to open mouth, neurologic signs, lysis of the tympanic bulla wall, and lysis within the temporal bone. However, only neurologic signs were shown to be a statistically significant predictor for the development of recurrence when using stepwise multivariable analysis.[1]

Of the neurologic signs reported by Greci and colleagues,[3] facial palsy and ataxia resolved after surgery, whereas preoperative head tilt persisted postoperatively.

Risk factors that were identified for recurrence or nonresolution of clinical signs were inability to open mouth in 19 cases (1 cured, 7 not cured), lysis of the bone of the tympanic bulla was present in 11 out of 18 cases imaged (4 cured, 7 not cured), expansion of the bulla was present in 11 out of 18 cases imaged (4 cured, 7 not cured), and bone lysis of the temporal bone was present in 6 out of 18 cases imaged (0 cured,

6 not cured). *Pseudomonas* was only cultured in cases that were not cured. Factors not associated with recurrence were osteoproliferation (6 out of 9 cured, 6 out of 9 not cured), lymph node enlargement (4 out of 9 cured, 3 out of 9 not cured).[1]

Of the dogs with recurrence reported by Greci and colleagues,[3] 2 were successfully treated (no recurrence at 32 and 42 months after second surgery). Two other dogs that had recurrence had a combination of multiple surgeries and continued medical management: one dog was treated surgically 4 times (LBO once, VBO 3 times) and still had persistent signs after the fourth surgery and one dog had 2 surgeries and medical management (antiinflammatory dose of steroids in conjunction with broad-spectrum antibiotics) after its second recurrence.[3]

Of the cases with recurrence described by Hardie and colleagues,[1] 3 of the 5 dogs with neurologic signs were euthanized without a revision surgery and 2 were managed with chronic systemic antibiotic therapy (one alive at the time of writing, one died of unrelated causes 29 months after the initial surgery). All 3 dogs presenting for inability or reluctance to open the mouth had a second surgery, and all required chronic intermittent systemic antibiotic therapy. Two died of unrelated causes at 37 and 40 months after the initial surgery, whereas the third was alive at the time of writing (52 months after the first surgery).[1]

SUMMARY

Surgical intervention can be curative. Dogs with early stage disease have a better outcome than dogs with more chronic disease and with temporal bone involvement.[1] Dogs with recurrent disease can be reoperated or managed medically with long-term resolution or palliation of clinical signs.

REFERENCES

1. Hardie EM, Linder KE, Pease AP. Aural cholesteatoma in twenty dogs. Vet Surg 2008;37(8):763–70.
2. Travetti O, Giudice C, Greci V, et al. Computed tomography features of middle ear cholesteatoma in dogs. Vet Radiol Ultrasound 2010;51(4):374–9.
3. Greci V, Travetti O, Di Giancamillo M, et al. Middle ear cholesteatoma in 11 dogs. Can Vet J 2011;52(6):631–6.
4. Schuenemann RM, Oechtering G. Cholesteatoma after lateral bulla osteotomy in two brachycephalic dogs. J Am Anim Hosp Assoc 2012;48(4):261–8.
5. Newman AW, Estey CM, McDonough S, et al. Cholesteatoma and meningoencephalitis in a dog with chronic otitis externa. Vet Clin Pathol 2015;44(1):157–63.
6. Olszewska E, Rutkowska J, Ozgirgin N. Consensus-based recommendations on the definition and classification of cholesteatoma. J Int Adv Otol 2015;11(1):81–7.
7. Little CJ, Lane JG, Gibbs C, et al. Inflammatory middle ear disease of the dog: the clinical and pathological features of cholesteatoma, a complication of otitis media. Vet Rec 1991;128(14):319–22.
8. Jackler RK, Santa Maria PL, Varsak YK, et al. A new theory on the pathogenesis of acquired cholesteatoma: mucosal traction. Laryngoscope 2015;125:S1–14.
9. Koizumi H, Suzuki H, Ikezaki S, et al. Osteoclasts are not activated in middle ear cholesteatoma. J Bone Miner Metab 2015. [Epub ahead of print].
10. Druss JG. Role which the epidermis plays in suppurations of the middle ear. Arch Otolaryngol 1933;17(4):484–502.
11. Schechter G. A review of cholesteatoma pathology. Laryngoscope 1969;79(11): 1907–20.

12. Uno Y, Satto R. Bone resorption in human cholesteatoma: morphological study with scanning electron microscopy. Ann Otol Rhinol Laryngol 1995;104(6):463–8.

13. Harran NX, Bradley KJ, Hetzel N, et al. MRI findings of a middle ear cholesteatoma in a dog. J Am Anim Hosp Assoc 2012;48(5):339–43.

14. Kemppainen HO, Puhakka HJ, Laippala PJ, et al. Epidemiology and aetiology of middle ear cholesteatoma. Acta Otolaryngol 1999;119(5):568–72.

15. Garosi LS, Dennis R, Schwarz T. Review of diagnostic imaging of ear diseases in the dog and cat. Vet Radiol Ultrasound 2003;44(2):137–46.

16. Doust R, King A, Hammond G, et al. Assessment of middle ear disease in the dog: a comparison of diagnostic imaging modalities. J Small Anim Pract 2007; 48(4):188–92.

17. Sturges BK, Dickinson PJ, Kortz GD, et al. Clinical signs, magnetic resonance imaging features, and outcome after surgical and medical treatment of otogenic intracranial infection in 11 cats and 4 dogs. J Vet Intern Med 2006;20(3):648–56.

18. Spivack RE, Elkins AD, Moore GE, et al. Postoperative complications following TECA-LBO in the dog and cat. J Am Anim Hosp Assoc 2013;49(3):160–8.

19. Davidson EB, Brodie HA, Breznock EM. Removal of a cholesteatoma in a dog, using a caudal auricular approach. J Am Vet Med Assoc 1997;211(12):1549–53.

20. Cohen MS, Landegger LD, Kozin ED, et al. Pediatric endoscopic ear surgery in clinical practice: lessons learned and early outcomes. Laryngoscope 2016; 126(3):732–8.

Current Treatment Options for Auricular Hematomas

Catriona MacPhail, DVM, PhD

KEYWORDS

- Ear • Pinna • Swelling • Drainage • Hematoma

KEY POINTS

- Aural hematomas most commonly occur due to self-trauma because of underlying ear disease.
- Benign neglect of aural hematomas results in permanent deformation of the pinna.
- Multiple management options exist to successfully address aural hematomas.
- Risk of recurrence is low, as long as underlying ear disease is well-controlled.

INTRODUCTION

Aural or auricular hematomas are fluctuant swellings filled with hemorrhagic fluid affecting the concave surface of the pinna in both dogs and cats (**Fig. 1**). This condition most commonly occurs as a result the shear forces created by violent head shaking or ear scratching secondary to otitis externa, yet some affected animals have no evidence of underlying ear disease. Bloody fluid accumulates under the skin of the inner pinna after vascular trauma and separation from the underlying cartilage. The exact location of the source of hemorrhage is not known but is thought to come from branches of the great auricular arteries and veins within, under, or between the cartilage layers. These vessels penetrate the scapha to supply the concave surface of the ear.

A separate theory with regard to cause involves underlying immunologic disease. A set of dogs and cats with aural hematomas were all found to have positive Coombs test in the serum and fluid retrieved from the pinna, although a small percentage had positive antinuclear antibodies (ANA) tests and identification of immunoglobulin G deposition at the dermoepidermal junction.[1] However, another study in dogs found none of the dogs with auricular hematomas were Coombs positive, or had positive ANA titers, although histopathological examination of biopsies showed evidence of an association with a hypersensitivity reaction.[2]

The author has nothing to disclose.
Department of Clinical Sciences, College of Veterinary Medicine and Biomedical Sciences, 1678 Campus Delivery, Colorado State University, Fort Collins, CO 80523-1678, USA
E-mail address: catriona.macphail@colostate.edu

Vet Clin Small Anim 46 (2016) 635–641
http://dx.doi.org/10.1016/j.cvsm.2016.01.003
0195-5616/16/$ – see front matter © 2016 Elsevier Inc. All rights reserved.

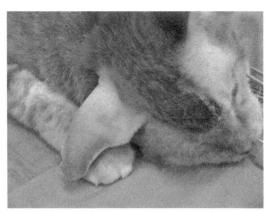

Fig. 1. A 3-year-old domestic shorthaired cat with a right aural hematoma secondary to scratching due to ear mite infestation.

PATIENT EVALUATION OVERVIEW

Aural hematomas can occur in dogs and cats of any breed or age, although dogs with long, pendulous ears may be more at risk. Animals should be evaluated for evidence of otitis externa, particularly looking for evidence of ear mite infestation (*Otodectes cynotis*) in cats. Because general anesthesia will be required for surgical treatment, routine bloodwork is typically indicated as an assessment of overall health.

TREATMENT OPTIONS

There are numerous techniques that have been described to address aural hematomas. Regardless, treatment of any underlying ear disease is crucial to minimize the chance of hematoma recurrence.

NONPHARMACOLOGIC TREATMENT OPTIONS

Without any specific aural hematoma treatment, secondary fibrosis and contraction will occur and can result in irreparable deformation of the pinna. Simple needle aspiration to drain the hematoma can be performed but recurrence is likely. When this pathway is chosen, daily drainage of the hematoma has been advocated to prevent early recurrence.[3] The concave surface of the pinna should be clipped and prepped before a large (16–20 g) hypodermic needle is inserted in the most dependent part of the pinna. Flushing with sterile saline can be performed to facilitate removal of clots and fibrin.

Other methods of drainage have been described with variable outcomes (**Box 1**). Typically, drains are inserted and secured on the concave (inner) surface of the pinna. A successful outcome in 5 dogs was described in a recent study in which active drains were inserted from the convex (outer) surface.[4]

PHARMACOLOGIC TREATMENT OPTIONS

The concurrent use of corticosteroids administered by different routes has been advocated with a variety of drainage and surgical treatments. Daily intravenous administration of dexamethasone (0.5–2.0 mg/kg) resulted in resolution in more than 85% of

---

Box 1
Methods of aural hematoma drainage

Teat cannula

Fenestrated silastic tubing

Penrose drain

Butterfly catheter (closed-suction drainage)

Data from Lanz OI, Wood BC. Surgery of the ear and pinna. Vet Clin North Am Small Anim Pract 2004;34:567–99.

---

cases.[5] Oral administration of anti-inflammatory doses of prednisone can help decrease head shaking and scratching, and may help treat inflammation associated with ear disease.[3] Injection of dexamethasone, methylprednisolone, and triamcinolone (**Box 2**) directly into the hematoma cavity following drainage of fluid has had successful resolution in more than 90% of cases.[5–7]

SURGICAL TREATMENT OPTIONS

The most common surgical method involves performing a curvilinear (S-shaped) incision in the concave surface of the pinna and placing full-thickness staggered longitudinal sutures throughout the pinna (**Fig. 2**):

1. After standard surgical clip and prep, the ear canal is filled with cotton balls or gauze to prevent fluid or hemorrhage from entering it.
2. A large S-shaped or curvilinear incision is made through the skin directly over the hematoma on the concave surface of the pinna (see **Fig. 2**A).
3. The pinna is massaged such that all the clots are removed.
4. The wound is flushed copiously with sterile saline to remove any clots or fibrin.
5. Multiple, staggered, full-thickness, interrupted mattress sutures, using monofilament, nonabsorbable suture material, are placed parallel to the long axis of the pinna throughout the entire hematoma region (see **Fig. 2**B). Sutures are placed such that the knots are located on the concave surface of the pinna. The author typically uses 2-0 to 3-0 polybutester or polypropylene on a straight cutting needle.

An alternative surgical technique has recently been described in 23 dogs.[8] Following creation of a longitudinal incision on the concave surface of the pinna, several suture lines (1–3) were placed intradermally parallel to and on either side of the incision, thereby avoiding any external sutures (**Fig. 3**A). Suture bites were placed

---

Box 2
Reported dosages of intralesional corticosteroids

Dexamethasone 0.2 to 0.4 mg in saline every 24 hours for 1 to 5 days

Methylprednisolone 0.5 to 1.0 mL every 7 days for 1 to 3 weeks

Triamcinolone 0.1 to 1.0 mL every 7 days for 1 to 3 weeks

Data from Refs.[5–7]

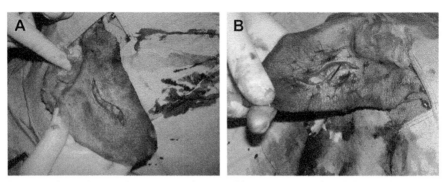

Fig. 2. Traditional surgical treatment of an aural hematoma in a dog. (*A*) An S-shaped incision is made on the concave surface of the pinna. (*B*) Multiple staggered sutures are placed parallel to the long axis of the pinna.

from the intradermal layer of the concave surface of the pinna to the cartilage (**Fig. 3**B). Monofilament absorbable suture (3-0 or 4-0 glycomer 631) was used to avoid the need for suture removal. No recurrence was documented in any of the 23 dogs and 91% had no auricular deformity. The advantages of this technique proposed by the investigators include minimal need for aftercare, absence of discomfort or irritation caused by external sutures, and lack of need for suture removal.

Other surgical techniques described involve the creation of circular fenestrations using either a 4 to 6 mm dermal biopsy punch or a carbon dioxide (CO_2) laser. When using a dermal punch, multiple partial-thickness circular plugs of tissue are removed approximately 1 to 1.5 cm apart from each other over the entire area of the hematoma.[9] The skin edge of each punch is tacked through the cartilage using a single simple interrupted suture of 3-0 to 4-0 monofilament suture.

The use of CO_2 laser has been described in 8 dogs.[10] In this technique, a 1 cm circular partial-thickness defect is created (into the hematoma only) in the most dependent part of the hematoma to facilitate drainage and flushing of the hematoma cavity. Multiple 1 to 2 mm full-thickness circular incisions were then made over the entire surface of the hematoma with the goal being to stimulate adhesion formation between the

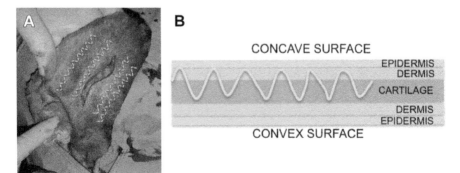

Fig. 3. Alterative internal suturing technique for aural hematomas. (*A*) 1 to 3 intradermal suture lines are placed parallel to the incision made in the concave surface of the pinna. (*B*) Longitudinal cross-section of the pinna, the continuous suture line is placed from concave dermis through the cartilage but not through to the convex surface.

cartilage layers due to fibrosis during cartilage healing. Outcomes and cosmetic appearance were reasonable, with no reports of hematoma recurrence.

A sutureless surgical technique for addressing aural hematomas is also available (Hematoma Repair System, Practivet, Phoenix, AZ, USA). Following the creation of the longitudinal incision on the concave surface of the pinna, preshaped silicon pads are placed on either side of the pinna. A needle is passed through the pad from medial to lateral facilitating placement of locking clips and rings over the entire surface of the ear (www.practivet.com). Pads are left on up to 3 weeks but daily inspection is required to observe for evidence of pressure necrosis.

POSTOPERATIVE CARE

Regardless of the technique used to address the hematoma, the use of a head bandage is controversial because maintaining a bandage can be difficult. However, if the ear hangs loose and the dog continues to shake its head, the repair is put under stress. At a minimum, an Elizabethan collar should be used in both dogs and cats to prevent self-trauma from scratching. Head bandages should be placed to allow access to the ear canal for appropriate treatment of underlying ear disease if indicated. The author prefers to secure the ear using a hematoma pad. The pad is secured to the ear using additional horizontal mattress sutures and left in place for 3 days. Hematoma pads are available commercially (Buster Othaematoma Compress, Kruuse Inc, Denmark) but they can also be made using simple materials found in most veterinary hospitals (**Box 3**, **Fig. 4**). Regardless of technique used, any external sutures should be left in place for a minimum of 3 weeks.

PROGNOSIS

Regardless of the mode of treatment, the likelihood of recurrence of aural hematoma is low as long as underlying ear disease is appropriately managed. There can be changes in the cosmetic appearance of the pinna; cats or dogs with erect or semierect ears may lose carriage of the pinna (**Fig. 5**).

Box 3
Aural hematoma pad

Materials (see Fig. 4A)

Piece of used radiographic film

Used surgical scrub brushes

Household cyanoacrylate (eg, Super Glue)

Technique

1. Remove the sponge from the scrub brush and split it in half to decrease the thickness of the sponge.

2. Trace the outline of the pinna on the piece of radiographic film.

3. Glue the sponges to the radiographic film to completely cover the outline of the pinna.

4. Once the glue has dried, cut along the trace of the pinna outline.

5. Attach the aural hematoma pad to the concave aspect of the pinna with 3 or 4 full-thickness mattress sutures (see **Fig. 4**B, C).

6. The pad is removed in 3 days. The remaining sutures are removed in 3 weeks (see **Fig. 4**D).

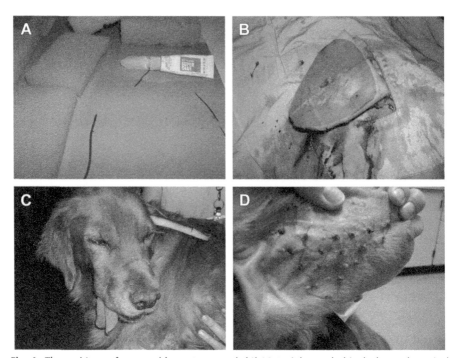

Fig. 4. The makings of an aural hematoma pad. (*A*) Materials needed include used surgical sponges, household cyanoacrylate glue, and used radiographic film. (*B*) The aural hematoma pad is attached directly to the concave aspect of the pinna with 3 to 4 full-thickness sutures. (*C*) The postoperative appearance following placement of an aural hematoma pad. (*D*) Appearance of the pinna following removal of the aural hematoma pad.

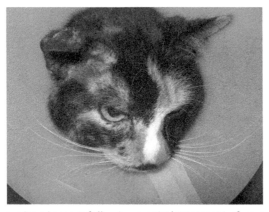

Fig. 5. Loss of ear carriage in a cat following surgical treatment of an aural hematoma.

REFERENCES

1. Kuwahara J. Canine and feline aural hematoma: clinical, experimental, and clinicopathologic observations. Am J Vet Res 1986;47:2300–8.
2. Joyce JA, Day MJ. Immunopathogenesis of canine aural haematoma. J Small Anim Pract 1997;38:152–8.
3. Lanz OI, Wood BC. Surgery of the ear and pinna. Vet Clin North Am Small Anim Pract 2004;34:567–99.
4. Pavletic MM. Use of laterally placed vacuum drains for management of aural hematomas in five dogs. J Am Vet Med Assoc 2015;246(1):112–7.
5. Kuwahara J. Canine and feline aural haematomas: results of treatment with corticosteroids. J Am Anim Hosp Assoc 1986;22:641–7.
6. Seibert R, Tobias KM. Surgical treatment for aural hematoma. NAVC Clinician's Brief 2013;3:29–32.
7. Romatowski J. Nonsurgical treatment of aural hematomas. J Am Vet Med Assoc 1994;204:1318.
8. Győrffy A, Szijártó A. A new operative technique for aural haematoma in dogs: a retrospective clinical study. Acta Vet Hung 2014;62:340–7.
9. Smeak DD. Surgery of the ear canal and pinna. In: Birchard SJ, Sherding RG, editors. Saunders manual of small animal practice. 3rd edition. St Louis (MO): Elsevier; 2006. p. 582–92.
10. Dye TL, Teague HD, Ostwald DA Jr, et al. Evaluation of a technique using the carbon dioxide laser for the treatment of aural hematomas. J Am Anim Hosp Assoc 2002;38:385–90.

Management of Otic and Nasopharyngeal, and Nasal Polyps in Cats and Dogs

Valentina Greci, DVM, PhD[a],*, Carlo Maria Mortellaro, DVM[b]

KEYWORDS

- Polyps • Aural • Otic • Nasopharyngeal • Nasal • Cat • Dog

KEY POINTS

- Feline inflammatory polyps are benign growths, which usually arise from the tympanic cavity or the eustachian tube.
- Diagnosis is based on clinical signs, diagnostic imaging, and histopathology; both minimally invasive and surgical techniques for polyp removal are effective.
- Feline nasal hamartomas are benign lesions that arise from the native tissues of the nasal cavity; despite their expansile behavior, they have a good prognosis after surgical or endoscopic removal.
- Inflammatory polyps are extremely rare in dogs; different polypoid-like masses have been described in the middle ear and nasal cavity in dogs, but these lesions likely have a different tissue origin than cats, and the outcome after removal is less consistently successful.

FELINE INFLAMMATORY POLYPS

Introduction

Feline inflammatory polyps (FIPs) are the most common nonneoplastic pedunculated growths found in the ear canal or nasopharynx in cats. They are presumed to originate from the epithelial lining of the tympanic bulla (aural inflammatory polyps) or the auditory tube. When they originate from the auditory tube, they can grow into the tympanic cavity (middle ear polyps) or the nasopharynx (nasopharyngeal polyps) or, less frequently, in both directions. Bilateral polyps have been reported but are uncommon.[1–14]

The cause of FIPs is still debated. It is unclear whether polyps are congenital in origin, or a response to an inflammatory process from chronic viral infection,

The authors have nothing to disclose.
[a] Internal Medicine and Endoscopy, Ospedale Veterinario Gregorio VII, Piazza di Villa Carpegna 52, Roma 00165, Italia; [b] Division of Small Animal Surgery, Department of Veterinary Medicine, Facoltà di Medicina Veterinaria, Università degli Studi di Milano, Via celoria 10, Milano 20133, Italia
* Corresponding author.
E-mail address: valentinagreci@gregoriovii.com

Vet Clin Small Anim 46 (2016) 643–661
http://dx.doi.org/10.1016/j.cvsm.2016.01.004
0195-5616/16/$ – see front matter © 2016 Elsevier Inc. All rights reserved.

or a consequence of chronic middle ear and/or upper respiratory inflammation.[2–4,7–10,14–21]

FIPs consist of a core of loosely arranged fibrovascular tissue covered by a stratified squamous or columnar epithelium. Inflammatory cells, primarily lymphocytes, plasma cells, and macrophages, are present within the stroma and are especially dense in the submucosal areas of the tissue. The mucosa is commonly ulcerated.[2,7–9,14,19,20]

Presumptive diagnosis of FIPs is based on history and physical examination, supported by imaging and endoscopic evaluation, and is confirmed by histopathological examination of biopsy samples.[7–10,13,14]

FIPs usually occur in young cats with an average age of 1.5 years, although they have been reported in cats of all ages.[2,4,7–9,14,20] The authors have diagnosed FIPs in Maine coon siblings and in 2 Maine coon cats from the same bloodline but from different environmental settings. There is some suggestion that because FIPs have been diagnosed in siblings, they may have a congenital origin.[22] FIPs in Maine coon cats might be inherited or congenital, or they might have a genetic predisposition to this condition.[22]

Clinical signs are usually progressive and chronic in nature. Aural inflammatory polyps usually result in chronic otitis externa, with cats most often exhibiting head shaking and otorrhea. Otic discharge can vary from waxy to purulent in nature.[9,13,14] When the polyp is visible within the ear canal, it has already protruded through a ruptured eardrum, and otitis media is frequently present.[9,10,16,17,20,23] Neurologic alterations, such as Horner syndrome, head tilt, ataxia, nystagmus, circling, and facial paralysis, may also be observed with middle and inner ear involvement.[2–5,7–11,13,14,16–20] The most common clinical signs in cats with nasopharyngeal polyps are nasal discharge, stertorous breathing, reverse sneezing, and sneezing.[2–9,11,16–20]

Other signs and related conditions associated with inflammatory polyps, such as dysphagia, megaesophagus, regurgitation, pulmonary hypertension, polyp abscess, submandibular swelling, suppurative meningoencephalitis, and severe dyspnea, have been rarely reported.[5,8,9,11,12,24–29]

Aural polyps can be seen on both conventional and video-otoscopy. In some cats, aural polyps can be directly seen protruding directly from the external ear canal.[2,8–10,14,24]

Nasopharyngeal polyps can be confirmed on digital palpation of the nasopharynx, rostral traction of the soft palate, or retrograde rhinoscopy.[2,7–9,14,20,24] Secondary otitis media is frequently present with nasopharyngeal polyps, because the mass occludes the auditory tube, resulting in mucous accumulation in the tympanic cavity.[2,8–10,17,20,23]

Imaging

Conventional radiology

Radiographs can be used to identify a soft tissue mass in the nasopharynx and to evaluate loss of the air contrast of the external ear canal and thickening of the tympanic bullae; when these signs are present, they are specific for the diagnosis of middle ear disease.[4,8,14,20,26,30–33] Nasopharyngeal polyps are usually observed on a standard lateral projection or obliqued lateral projections (**Fig. 1**).[20,26,31,33]

In cats, the tympanic cavity is unequally divided into 2 compartments by a thin bony septum, giving it a double-chambered appearance. On plain radiographs, the best images to view the tympanic bullae are right and left lateral oblique and the rostrocaudal projections. In these views, normal bullae appear as thin-walled, air-filled rounded structures at the base of the skull (**Fig. 2**). The rostrocaudal projections are particularly

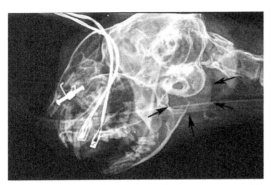

Fig. 1. Pharyngeal soft tissue density in 30° lateral view of a cat with a nasopharyngeal polyp (*black arrows*).

useful to evaluate both the tympanic bullae and the horizontal ear canals.[30,31,33–35] Dorsoventral and ventrodorsal projections are less diagnostic due to partial superimposition of the petrous temporal bone over the bullae.[30,33]

Radiographic changes that are often evident in cats with otic polyps include loss of air contrast in the ear canal and/or the tympanic bulla, tympanic bone thickening, and

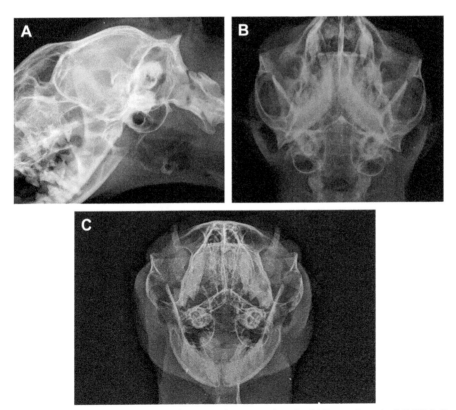

Fig. 2. Radiographic appearance of a normal ear canal and middle ear in cats: (*A*) 30° left lateral, (*B*) rostro 10° ventrocaudodorsal, (*C*) rostroventral-caudodorsal open mouth views.

the presence of a soft tissue mass in the pharynx or ear canal; sclerosis noted within the petrous bone may suggest otitis interna (**Fig. 3**).[14,26,30,31,33] Some cats with FIPs have normal plain radiographs; the diagnosis of FIPs in these instances is often substantiated with endoscopic examination or advanced imaging modalities.[14,26,30,31,33]

Computed tomography

Computed tomography (CT) allows cross-sectional imaging of the external, middle, and internal parts of the ear and nasopharynx. Skull positioning should be precise to allow comparison of symmetry; CT imaging has the advantage of allowing image reformatting in various planes, eliminating superimposition of surrounding boney structures. In addition, CT imaging shows good soft tissue contrast resolution.[8,20,26,30,31,33]

CT allows evaluation of fluid or tissue within the external and/or the tympanic cavity, changes in the tympanic bulla contour, presence/absence of bony proliferation, and/or evidence of osteolysis. Thin slicing provides great anatomic detail of middle ear and inner ear structures.[30,31] CT is more specific in localizing the affected osseous bulla and earlier detection of small masses of both the tympanic cavity and the nasopharynx. Therefore, because of these advantages, CT imaging is superior to conventional radiography and thus allows more specific prognosis and treatment planning for cats with suspected tympanic masses.[30,33]

On CT, FIPs typically appear as an oval homogenous space-occupying dense structure with well-defined borders and hard rim enhancement (**Fig. 4**).[26-30,36] More aggressive infections and neoplastic conditions often exhibit both osteoproliferative and lytic lesions of the tympanic bulla. On contrast CT images, these aggressive conditions exhibit marked contrast medium enhancement compared with FIPs in cats.[27,30,31,36]

MRI

Only a few reports mention the use of MRI in the diagnosis of feline ear diseases. Similar to cats with FIPs, other inflammatory middle ear diseases are often characterized by contrast enhancement along the inner margin of the tympanic bulla due to the presence of vascularized tissue lining this region. Unless osteoproliferative and/or lytic

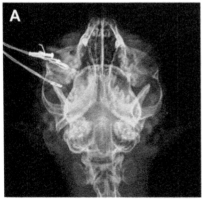 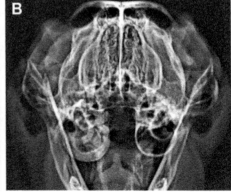

Fig. 3. Different radiographic appearances of middle ear polyps in cats: (*A*) loss of air contrast within the bulla and the ear canal and mild thickening of the right bulla contour; (*B*) mild bulla enlargement, severe thickening of the bulla contour and septum, erosion of the petrous bone, loss of air contrast within the right bulla and the ear canal.

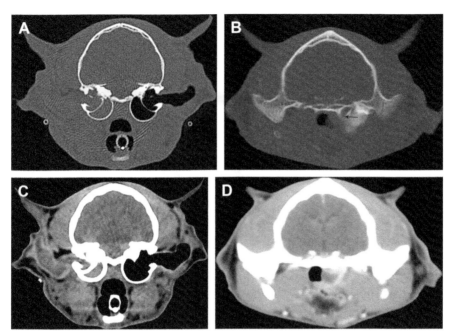

Fig. 4. CT appearance of FIPs. (*A*) Bone tissue window (BTW): the middle ear cavity and ipsilateral ear canal are filled with a homogenous soft tissue dense structure. (*B*) BTW: a soft tissue density is partially filling the nasopharynx, and there is ipsilateral eustachian tube enlargement (*black arrow*). (*C, D*) STW after contrast medium administration in the same cat: the lesion appears as an oval homogenous space-occupying soft tissue dense structure with well-defined borders and contrast rim enhancement. (*Courtesy of* [*C* and *D*] Dr Simone Borgonovo, Clinica Veterinaria Gran Sasso, Milano, Italia.)

changes are evident in the tympanic bulla, it can be difficult to differentiate an inflammatory polyp from inflammatory tissue from otitis media, or early neoplastic conditions within the tympanic cavity.[8,20,29–31,37,38] However, MRI is indicated in cats presenting with concurrent peripheral nerve and central nervous system disease to better evaluate the inner ear and surrounding neural structures when more aggressive lesions are suspected.[26,29]

Endoscopy
When evaluating cats with FIPs, both ear canals and nasopharynx should be examined with endoscopy.

The presence of thick waxy cerumen or purulent exudate is often noted on otoscopy. After ear canal cleaning, aural polyps usually appear as pink pale to reddish rounded, sometimes multilobulated or ulcerated masses in the ear canal or within the tympanic cavity (**Fig. 5**).[9,10,14] When a mass is observed that does not appear as an FIP, fine-needle biopsy or pinch biopsy may be indicated first to achieve a definitive diagnosis, and for appropriate treatment planning (see **Fig. 5**D).[14,39]

A thickened opaque or bulging eardrum on the contralateral side is often seen due to impairment of auditory tube drainage secondary to nasopharyngeal inflammation or pressure from the nasopharyngeal polyp. If a small polyp arising just behind a bulging tympanum is suspected, a myringotomy can be performed to explore the tympanic cavity (**Fig. 6**).

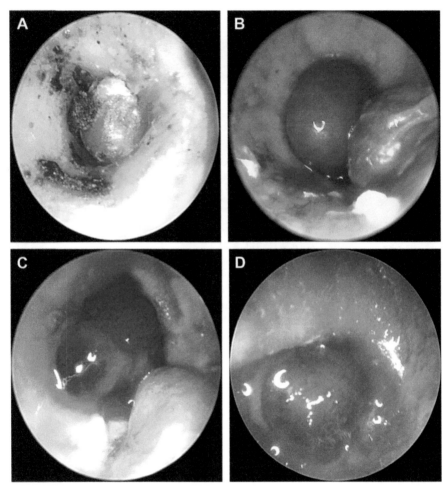

Fig. 5. Different endoscopic appearances of aural inflammatory polyps: (*A*) polyp protruding behind the tympanum; (*B*) polyp protruding through a ruptured tympanum, portion of the tympanum is still visible on the right; (*C*) multilobulated ulcerated polyp; (*D*) oval pink highly vascularized polyp, given the aspect the mass was biopsied for final diagnosis.

Nasopharyngeal polyps can be seen endoscopically or by rostrally displacing the soft palate with a hooked instrument such as a spay hook (**Fig. 7**).

Treatment

Both minimally invasive and traditional surgical techniques have been described to remove FIPs.

Minimally invasive approach

Traction/avulsion of polyps Traction/avulsion is the simplest form of treatment, without requiring specialized equipment. The polyp is generally grasped with a toothed grasping forceps (curved clamp, Allis, or alligator forceps), and removed by firm traction with rotation until the polyp detaches at the stalk.[2,3,7–10,17,20,24]

Aural polyps are removed by positioning the cat in lateral recumbency after routine preparation of the ear. Removal of multilobulated polyps can be difficult because they

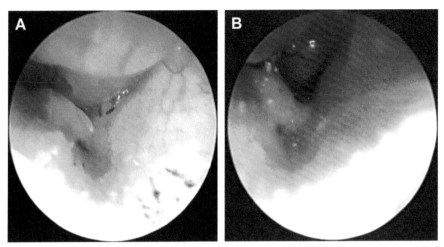

Fig. 6. Otoscopic views of a cat with an aural inflammatory polyp. (*A*) Severe tympanum bulging is shown before myringotomy; (*B*) a small middle ear polyp is evident after myringotomy.

tend to rupture and bleed from the cut surface of the mass; repeated grasping and pulling may be necessary to debulk the mass. In this instance, a portion of the stalk remnant may remain, which increases the risk of polyp recurrence. Increased exposure can be obtained by performing a lateral ear canal resection, but this is rarely necessary.[7,9,10,17,20,24]

Nasopharyngeal polyps are removed by placing the cat in dorsal recumbency; the polyp can be visualized by application of digital pressure on the rostral soft palate, displacing the mass caudally, or by retracting the palate rostrally with a spay hook or preplaced stay sutures in the terminal aspect of the soft palate (**Fig. 8**). Additional exposure can be achieved by performing a direct incision through the soft palate midline directly over the polyp, but this is rarely necessary. If a staphylotomy is elected, attempt to leave the distal 5 mm of the palate intact to help avoid incisional dehiscence after surgery. Retracting the edges of the incision with stay sutures can help provide additional exposure. The soft palate is repaired in 2 layers with absorbable suture.[2–5,7–10,18,20,24]

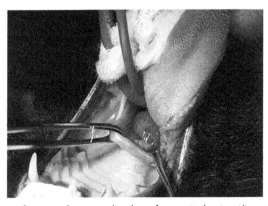

Fig. 7. Visualization of a nasopharyngeal polyp after rostral retraction of the soft palate.

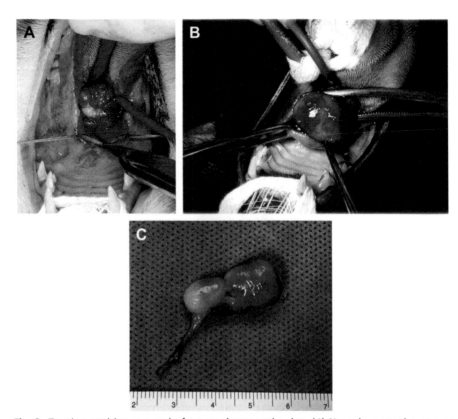

Fig. 8. Traction-avulsion removal of a nasopharyngeal polyp. (*A*) Nasopharyngeal exposure can be obtained by use of anatomic forceps/clamp or gentle traction by stay sutures (shown). (*B*) The polyp is then grasped and pulled with hemostatic forceps until the stalk detaches. (*C*) A 3-cm oval, pale pink bilobated nasopharyngeal polyp with stalk attached; note the long stalk that was originating and filling the Eustachian tube.

Minor to moderate hemorrhage is expected following these traction/avulsion of nasopharyngeal polyps, but the bleeding generally stops spontaneously, or after applying dorsal pressure to the palatine area for several minutes.[10,14]

Endoscopic removal of polyps Recently a per-endoscopic transtympanic traction (PTT) removal technique has been described.[14] After cleaning the ear and positioning the patient in lateral recumbency, the polyp is grasped under direct endoscopic visualization with an endoscopic forceps and pulled with a rotating movement until the polyp is detached.

After removal, soft tissue or remnants of the polyp "footprint" within the tympanic cavity are curetted under direct endoscopic visualization with a Volkmann spoon or otologic spoon (**Fig. 9**). When necessary, the septum that separates the feline double-chambered tympanic cavity is removed using a pinch biopsy forceps under endoscopic visualization. Hemorrhage is usually mild, and it is easily controlled by flushing with sterile refrigerated 0.9% NaCl solution.[14]

Laser ablation of polyps Carbon dioxide laser ablation of polyps is another promising technique for aural polyp removal. This technique is performed under visualization with

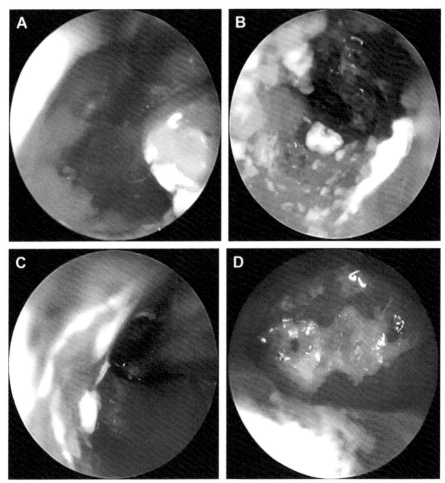

Fig. 9. Step-by-step endoscopic images of PTT procedure: (*A*) grasping of the polyp in tympanic cavity via endoscope; (*B*) appearance after polyp removal with remnant tissue in upper right region of tympanic cavity; (*C*) use of an otologic spoon during endoscopic curettage; (*D*) bone surface of tympanic cavity after endoscopic curettage of remaining soft tissue remnants.

a video-otoscope. A special rigid laser tip, 120 mm long, is placed through the 2-mm working channel of a dedicated video-otoscope. Smaller polyps can be debulked by direct laser vaporization of the polyp; charred tissue is then removed by irrigation. This laser procedure is repeated until the stalk of the polyp is no longer visualized.

With larger polyps, the tip of the laser is pushed into the tympanic cavity along the floor of the horizontal ear canal under the polyp mass; laser energy is then applied to vaporize the entire polyp, or it can be partially removed to facilitate traction removal. Afterward, the laser tip is placed into the bulla cavity toward the residual stalk, and laser energy is applied until the stalk is no longer visible.[10,20]

Open surgical removal
Ventral bulla osteotomy (VBO) has been proposed by veterinary surgeons as the treatment of choice for FIPs because of the high incidence of concurrent middle ear

involvement.[4,7–10,13,16,19,20,32,40–42] Because the cat has a double-chambered tympanic cavity, VBO allows full exploration of both chambers by breeching the septum that separates the 2 compartments.[10,14,24]

Some investigators suggest VBO even in the absence of radiographic middle ear involvement[20,40–42]; some other investigators recommend VBO to improve the outcome and reduce the risk of recurrence in cats affected only by nasopharyngeal polyp.[8,11,18,41] Prospective clinical trials with randomized minimally invasive versus open surgical treatment of FIPs are needed to help determine the best approach for cats with FIPs.

Cats presenting with a nasopharyngeal or aural polyp may show signs of middle ear disease even with no radiographic evidence of an ear polyp or otitis media; these signs are thought to occur because of inflammation secondary to pressure changes and mucous accumulation within the tympanic cavity. This condition usually resolves after minimally invasive techniques of polyp removal and postoperative corticosteroid administration.[23] In these cases, open surgical removal has been questioned, and minimally invasive approaches are recommended for polyp removal. VBO is more invasive and has higher morbidity than traction/avulsion with or without lateral ear canal resection or incision of the soft palate or PTT.[7,10]

According to the authors' experience, VBO should be considered only when polyps recur more than twice in a short period after traction avulsion through a minimally invasive approach.

VBO may be indicated in cats that have mild to moderate stenosis of the horizontal ear canal. This stenosis would limit curettage of the mucosa lining the tympanic cavity via PTT or after lateral ear canal resection.

Total ear canal ablation and lateral bulla osteotomy (TECALBO) is usually indicated for more invasive ear conditions; however, few chronic cases of FIPs might show severe stenosis of the horizontal ear canal or adhesions to the ear wall canal, thus not enabling extirpation of the polyp. For these cases, TECALBO might represent the best surgical technique.[13,43,44]

Complications and polyp recurrence among different techniques after polyp removal Regardless of the polyp removal technique, postoperative complications, such as Horner syndrome, vestibular syndrome, facial nerve paralysis, chronic otitis media, and interna, can occur; these complications can be temporary or permanent.[7–11,14,18,20,40–42]

Minimally invasive approaches for polyp removal are preferred because complications are less common than with open surgical approaches. Horner syndrome was less frequent in cats treated by PTT (8%) than in cats treated by VBO (57%–95%) or by traction alone (43%). In some cats treated by VBO, Horner syndrome can be permanent. Temporary and permanent facial nerve paralysis has been reported with VBO and TECALBO, but not with traction alone or PTT.[7–11,14,19,20,40–44]

Otitis media is frequently associated with FIPS; postoperative antibiotic therapy should be administered to treat concurrent and prevent secondary otitis media, and the antibiotics should be chosen based on culture and susceptibility tests.[7–9,14,20,23] Chronic otitis media can be a long-term complication after polyp removal. In a series of cats treated by PTT, 2 cats (5.4%) had ongoing chronic otitis media as a long-term complication. The frequency of otitis media after polyp removal in other case series has not been well recorded.[7,9,14,20,23,24]

Polyp recurrence has been reported to occur from 19 days to 46 months postoperatively with all the techniques mentioned to remove FIPs.[7–10,14] Recurrence in cats treated by simple traction was frequent when there was evidence of middle ear radiographic involvement.[7] The percentage of recurrence for PTT (13.5%) reported is lower than the ones reported for traction alone (33%–57%) and similar to the percentages reported for VBO (0%–33%).[7–11,14,19,20,25,40,41] The lower recurrence rate reported for VBO and PTT is due to the more complete extirpation of the mucosa lining the tympanic cavity compared with simple traction.[9,10,14,24,42]

Recurrence rate for simple traction might be reduced by curetting the mucosa lining the tympanic cavity with an otologic spoon after traction avulsion of polyps. Polyp recurrence and postoperative complication rates following laser ablation have not been reported.

FELINE INFLAMMATORY POLYPS OF THE NASAL TURBINATES (HAMARTOMA)

Inflammatory polyps of the nasal turbinates was a terminology used to describe a different polypoid-like benign growth of the nasal cavity in cats, which was once considered to be a rare manifestation of nasopharyngeal polyps.[13,45,46] However, it has been recently reported that the histopathological appearance of these lesions resembles the human chondromesenchymal hamartoma characterized by fibrovascular tissue lined by a stratified squamous or ciliated columnar epithelium and bony-cartilage structures without signs of atypia and erythrocytes-filled spaces.[13,47]

Feline nasal chondromesenchymal hamartomas (FNCMH) should be considered a separate entity, because they arise from the native tissue of the nasal cavities rather than the eustachian tube or tympanic cavity.[13,47]

The condition, originally thought to be encountered more often in Italy, was once thought to be related to genetic or environmental factor. The disease is now rarely diagnosed. Sporadic cases have been reported in the United States, and one case was cited in the United Kingdom.[45–47]

The disease is usually diagnosed in young cats without any known breed predisposition. Cats present with progressive stertorous breathing, sneezing, open-mouth breathing, serous nasal discharge, epiphora, and epistaxis. In severe cases, cats have sinonasal deformation or a mass lesion protruding from the nostrils.[13,45–47]

Radiographic studies typically demonstrate soft tissue opacification of the nasal cavity, turbinate lysis, and radiolucent areas, corresponding to cystic spaces within the lesion.[13,46,47] CT features of FNCMH are shown in **Fig. 10**. Turbinate and bone loss is likely to be secondary to compression atrophy given the expansile but noninfiltrative behavior of these masses.

Endoscopically, the lesion appears as a multilobulated pink to bluish lesion occupying the nasopharynx and the nasal cavities; pinch biopsies collected endoscopically must be submitted for histopathological examination to achieve a definite diagnosis.[47]

Although spontaneous regression has been reported as well as response to corticosteroid treatment, it has been recommended that these masses be removed, endoscopically, or for more extensive lesions, by rhinotomy, to facilitate complete excision.[13,46,47]

Despite the potential expansile and seemingly destructive behavior of chondromesenchymal hamartomas, this disease usually has a good prognosis, and recurrence after treatment has been rarely reported.[13,47]

CANINE POLYPS
Introduction

Canine ear and nasopharyngeal polyps are rare and generally unilateral, but few have been reported bilaterally.[9,10,48–50]

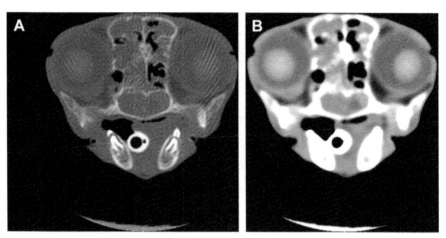

Fig. 10. CT aspects of FNCMH: (*A*) BTW at the level of temporomandibular joint: a soft tissue dense mass is shown filling the nasopharynx and right sinonasal cavities, and partially filling the left sinonasal cavities; turbinate loss and rarefaction are also visible; (*B*) STW after contrast medium administration: note the patchy contrast enhancement.

Clinicians must be aware that the definition of inflammatory polyp represents a macroscopic description of a pedunculated to grossly lobulated lesion that histologically is considered benign.

Macroscopic evidence of a polypoid-like lesion in the nasopharynx or in the ear in dogs likely is different in character than typical inflammatory polyps in cats.

The definition of inflammatory polyp should be restricted to those lesions that resemble the feline and human counterpart as described for the well-known otic and nasopharyngeal inflammatory polyps and should not comprise keratinizing epithelium.[7–11,51–54]

Aural polyps
Inflammatory polyps arising from the ear canal wall can be removed with the narrow attachment by simple traction, or they can be removed with surgical excision (**Fig. 11**); they might recur as described in cats.

Canine aural polyps should not be confused with ceruminous gland adenomas; adenomas might grossly look like a polypoid growth, but they cannot be removed by traction because they have a broad attachment to the ear canal skin.[10]

In dogs, cholesterol granulomas, cholesteatomas, and proliferative otitis media can be mistaken for polyps, so histologic confirmation before contemplating mass removal is important.[23,55–61]

Clinical presentation is usually characterized by otorrhea, ear scratching, and head shaking, and clinical signs of otitis media/interna are frequently present; diagnostic imaging also differs from FIPs (**Figs. 12** and **13**).[10,30,31,55–67] Treatment and prognosis depend on histologic diagnosis (**Fig. 14**); however, surgical removal via VBO or TECALBO is often necessary.[10,55–60]

Nasal and nasopharyngeal polyps
Canine nasal and nasopharyngeal polyps that histologically resemble the feline and human inflammatory polyps should be treated as described for inflammatory polyps in cats.[49,50,54] Different nasal hamartomas have been described in dogs, which

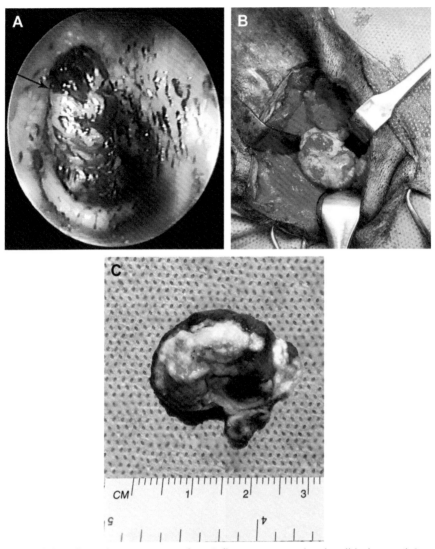

Fig. 11. (A) Endoscopic appearance of an inflammatory aural polyp (black arrow) in a 5-year-old female spayed Belgian shepherd presenting with chronic otitis externa; (B) surgical exposure of a recurrent polyp of the horizontal ear canal protruding into the tympanic cavity in a 6-year-old English Bull Dog during total ear canal ablation and lateral bulla ostetomy; (C) macroscopic appearance of the aural polyp removed surgically: a 2-cm oval irregular pale yellowish aural polyp with a short stalk.

macroscopically look like a polypoid mass. Histopathologically, they are characterized by connective tissue with inflammatory cells infiltrates, and they do not show any evidence of neoplasia and are thought to arise from native tissue of the nasopharyngeal cavities.[47,68–74]

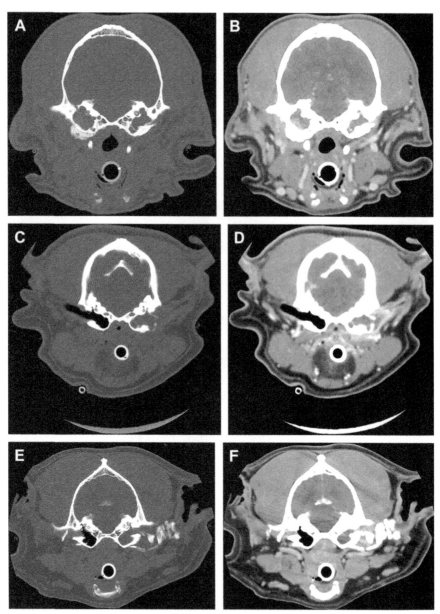

Fig. 12. CT imaging of canine middle ear polypoid-like lesions. (*A*) BTW: the right bulla is slightly enlarged and filled with a soft tissue density in the tympanic cavity; moderate thickening and mottled lysis of the bulla, erosion of the petrous bone, and temporal-mandibular joint thickening are visible. The left bulla is filled by the same soft tissue density; note the mild thickening of the bulla contour and minimal petrous bone erosion. There is bilateral loss of air contrast of the ear canal. (*B*) Soft tissue window (STW) after contrast medium administration (acma): minimal contrast enhancement is bilateral. The dog was diagnosed with bilateral cholesteatoma. (*C*) BTW: a soft tissue density is filling the right tympanic cavity and protruding into the ear canal; mild enlargement of the tympanic bulla, mild thickening of the bulla contour, and loss of air contrast of the horizontal ear canal are also visible.

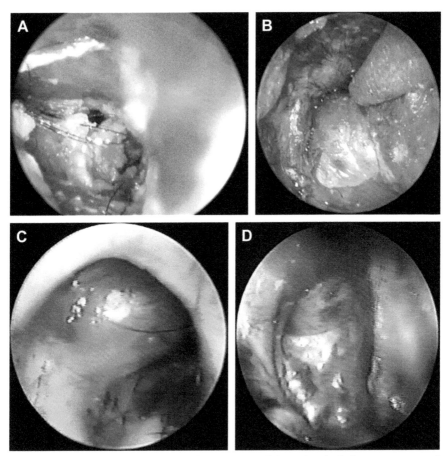

Fig. 13. Polypoid-like lesion of the middle ear cavity of dogs. (*A*, *B*) Cholesteatomas: pearly lesion to pink oval mass protruding from the middle ear. (*C*) Cholesterol granuloma: pink bluish oval lesion protruding from the middle ear cavity. (*D*) Otitis media: mass lesion filling the middle ear cavity.

CT appearance of the reported cases of canine polyps resembles nasal hamartomas.[68–71] Treatment planning depends on the definitive diagnosis; endoscopic or surgical intervention may be considered and full excision is often curative.[68–71]

Recently, neoplastic transformation of adenomatoidchondro-osseous nasal hamartoma has been described in humans; therefore, prompt diagnosis and treatment should be considered to avoid possible neoplastic transformation of a chronic benign disease.[75]

(*D*) STW acma: heterogenous contrast enhancement. The dog was diagnosed with cholesterol granuloma. (*E*) BTW: loss of air contrast in the left tympanic cavity and ear canal, thickening and calcification of the external ear canal; loss of air contrast of the right external ear. (*F*) STW acma: minimal contrast enhancement of the left external ear canal. The dog was diagnosed with chronic otitis externa and chronic left otitis media.

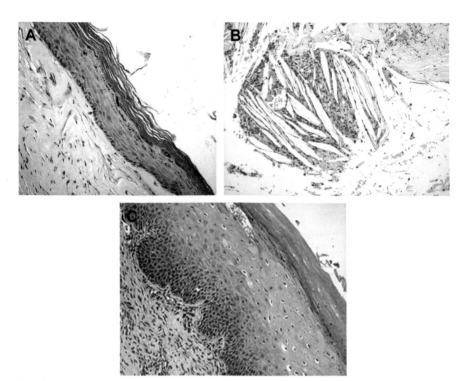

Fig. 14. Microscopic appearance of (*A*) cholesteatoma: presence of a hyperplastic and hyperkeratotic keratinizing squamous epithelium lining a cystic cavity filled with keratin debris and resting on a dense fibrous stroma (hematoxylin and eosin [H&E], ×100). (*B*) Cholesterol granuloma: fibroconnective tissue, subepithelial inflammatory infiltration, areas of hemorrhages, and cholesterol cleft (H&E, ×100). (*C*) Otitis media: fibrovascular tissue with subepithelial inflammatory infiltration lined by a simple epithelium (H&E, ×100). (*Courtesy of* Dr Chiara Giudice, Università Veterinaria di Milano, Milano, Italia.)

REFERENCES

1. Harvey CE, Goldschmidt MH. Inflammatory polypoid growths in the ear canal of cats. J Small Anim Pract 1978;19:669–77.

2. Lane JG, Orr CM, Lucke VM, et al. Nasopharyngeal polyps arising in the middle ear of the cat. J Small Anim Pract 1981;22:511–22.

3. Bedford PG, Coulson A, Sharp NJ, et al. Nasopharyngeal polyps in the cat. Vet Rec 1981;109:551–3.

4. Bradley RL. Selected oral, pharyngeal, and upper respiratory conditions in the cat. Oral tumors, nasopharyngeal and middle ear polyps, and chronic rhinitis and sinusitis. Vet Clin North Am Small Anim Pract 1984;14:1173–84.

5. Brownlie SE, Bedford PG. Nasopharyngeal polyp in a kitten. Vet Rec 1985;117:668–9.

6. Pope ER. Feline inflammatory polyps. Semin Vet Med Surg (Small Anim) 1995;10: 87–93.

7. Anderson DM, Robinson RK, White RA. Management of inflammatory polyps in 37 cats. Vet Rec 2000;147:684–7.

8. Kudnig ST. Nasopharyngeal polyps in cats. Clin Tech Small Anim Pract 2002;17: 174–7.

9. Fan TM, de Lorimier LP. Inflammatory polyps and aural neoplasia. Vet Clin North Am Small Anim Pract 2004;34:489–509.
10. Gotthelf LN. Inflammatory polyps. In: Gotthelf LN, editor. Small animal ear diseases, an illustrated guide. St Louis (MO): Elsevier Saunders; 2005. p. 317–28.
11. MacPhail CM, Innocenti CM, Kudnig ST, et al. Atypical manifestations of feline inflammatory polyps in three cats. J Feline Med Surg 2007;9:219–25.
12. Anders BB, Hoelzler MG, Scavelli TD, et al. Analysis of auditory and neurologic effects associated with ventral bulla osteotomy for removal of inflammatory polyps or nasopharyngeal masses in cats. J Am Vet Med Assoc 2008;233:580–5.
13. Reed N, Gunn-Moore D. Nasopharyngeal disease in cats: 2. Specific conditions and their management. J Feline Med Surg 2012;14:317–26.
14. Greci V, Vernia E, Mortellaro CM. Per-endoscopic trans-tympanic traction for the management of feline aural inflammatory polyps: a case review of 37 cats. J Feline Med Surg 2014;16:645–50.
15. Baker G. Nasopharyngeal polyps in cats. Vet Rec 1982;111:43.
16. Parker NR, Binnington AG. Nasopharyngeal polyps in cats: three case reports and a review of the literature. J Am Anim Hosp Assoc 1985;21:473–8.
17. Norris AM, Laing EJ. Diseases of the nose and sinuses. Vet Clin North Am Small Anim Pract 1985;15:865–90.
18. Landsborough L. Nasopharyngeal polyp in a five-month-old Abyssinian kitten. Can Vet J 1994;35:383–4.
19. Veir JK, Lappin MR, Foley JE, et al. Feline inflammatory polyps: historical, clinical, and PCR findings for feline calici virus and feline herpes virus-1 in 28 cases. J Feline Med Surg 2002;4:195–9.
20. Muilenburg RK, Fry TR. Feline nasopharyngeal polyps. Vet Clin North Am Small Anim Pract 2002;32:839–49.
21. Klose TC, MacPhail CM, Schultheiss PC, et al. Prevalence of select infectious agents in inflammatory aural and nasopharyngeal polyps from client-owned cats. J Feline Med Surg 2010;12:769–74.
22. Stanton ME, Wheaton LG, Render JA, et al. Pharyngeal polyps in two feline siblings. J Am Vet Med Assoc 1985;186:1311–3.
23. Gotthelf LN. Diagnosis and treatment of otitis media in dogs and cats. Vet Clin North Am Small Anim Pract 2004;34:469–87.
24. Lanz OI, Wood BC. Surgery of the ear and pinna. Vet Clin North Am Small Anim Pract 2004;34:567–99.
25. Byron JK, Shadwick SR, Bennett AR. Megaesophagus in a 6-month-old cat secondary to a nasopharyngeal polyp. J Feline Med Surg 2010;12:322–4.
26. Fazio CG, Dennison SE, Forrest LJ. What is your diagnosis? Nasopharyngeal polyp. J Am Vet Med Assoc 2011;239:187–8.
27. Rosenblatt AJ, Zito SJ, Webster NS. What is your diagnosis? Unilateral inflammatory polyp. J Am Vet Med Assoc 2014;244:37–9.
28. Pilton JL, Ley CJ, Voss K, et al. Atypical abscessated nasopharyngeal polyp associated with expansion and lysis of the tympanic bulla. J Feline Med Surg 2014;16:699–702.
29. Cook LB, Bergman RL, Bahr A, et al. Inflammatory polyp in the middle ear with secondary suppurative meningoencephalitis in a cat. Vet Radiol Ultrasound 2003;44:648–51.
30. Garosi LS, Dennis R, Schwarz T. Review of diagnostic imaging of ear diseases in the dog and cat. Vet Radiol Ultrasound 2003;44:137–46.
31. Bischoff MG, Kneller SK. Diagnostic imaging of the canine and feline ear. Vet Clin North Am Small Anim Pract 2004;34:437–58.

32. Boothe HW. Surgery of the tympanic bulla (otitis media and nasopharyngeal polyps). Probl Vet Med 1991;3:254–69.
33. Reed N, Gunn-Moore D. Nasopharyngeal disease in cats: 1. Diagnostic investigation. J Feline Med Surg 2012;14:306–15.
34. Hofer P, Meisen N, Bartholdi S, et al. A new radiographic view of the feline tympanic bullae. Vet Radiol Ultrasound 1995;36:14–5.
35. Hammond GJ, Sullivan M, Weinrauch S, et al. A comparison of the rostrocaudal open mouth and rostro 10 degrees ventro-caudodorsal oblique radiographic views for imaging fluid in the feline tympanic bulla. Vet Radiol Ultrasound 2005; 46:205–9.
36. Oliveira CR, O'Brien RT, Matheson JS, et al. Computed tomographic features of feline nasopharyngeal polyps. Vet Radiol Ultrasound 2012;53:406–11.
37. Allgoewer I, Lucas S, Schmitz SA. Magnetic resonance imaging of the normal and diseased feline middle ear. Vet Radiol Ultrasound 2000;41:413–8.
38. Sturges BK, Dickinson PJ, Kortz GD, et al. Clinical signs, magnetic resonance imaging features, and outcome after surgical and medical treatment of otogenic intracranial infection in 11 cats and 4 dogs. J Vet Intern Med 2006;20:648–56.
39. De Lorenzi D, Bonfanti U, Masserdotti C, et al. Fine-needle biopsy of external ear canal masses in the cat: cytologic results and histologic correlations in 27 cases. Vet Clin Pathol 2005;34:100–5.
40. Faulkner JE, Budsberg SC. Results of ventral bulla osteotomy for treatment of middle ear polyps in cats. J Am Vet Med Assoc 1990;26:496–9.
41. Kapatkin AS, Matthiesen DT. Results of surgery and long-term follow-up in 31 cats with nasopharyngeal polyps. J Am Anim Hosp Assoc 1990;26:387–92.
42. Trevor PB, Martin RA. Tympanic bulla osteotomy for treatment of middle-ear disease in cats: 19 cases (1984-1991). J Am Vet Med Assoc 1993;202:123–8.
43. Williams JM, White RAS. Total ear canal ablation combined with lateral bulla osteotomy in the cat. J Small Anim Pract 1992;5:225–7.
44. Bacon NJ, Gilbert RL, Bostock DE, et al. Total ear canal ablation in the cat: indications, morbidity and long-term survival. J Small Anim Pract 2003 Oct;44(10): 430–4.
45. Carpenter JL, Andrews LK, Holzworth J. Tumors and tumor-like lesions. In: Holzworth J, editor. Disease of the cat. Philadelphia: WB Saunders; 1987. p. 406–596.
46. Galloway PE, Kyles A, Henderson JP. Nasal polyps in a cat. J Small Anim Pract 1997;38:78–80.
47. Greci V, Mortellaro CM, Olivero D, et al. Inflammatory polyps of the nasal turbinates of cats: an argument for designation as feline mesenchymal nasal hamartoma. J Feline Med Surg 2011;13:213–9.
48. London CA, Dubilzeig RR, Vail DM, et al. Evaluation of dogs and cats with tumors of the ear canal: 145 cases (1978-1992). J Am Vet Med Assoc 1996;208:1413–8.
49. Billen F, Day MJ, Clercx C. Diagnosis of pharyngeal disorders in dogs: a retrospective study of 67 cases. J Small Anim Pract 2006;47:122–9.
50. Lobetti RG. A retrospective study of chronic nasal disease in 75 dogs. J S Afr Vet Assoc 2009;80:224–8.
51. Seitz SE, Losonsky JM, Maretta SM. Computed tomographic appearance of inflammatory polyps in three cats. Vet Radiol Ultrasound 1996;37:99–104.
52. Thompson LD. Otic polyp. Ear Nose Throat J 2012;91:474–5.
53. Newton JR, Ah-See KW. A review of nasal polyposis. Ther Clin Risk Manag 2008; 4:507–12.

54. Fingland RB, Gratzek A, Vorhies MW, et al. Nasopharyngeal polyp in a dog. J Am Anim Hosp Assoc 1993;29:311–4.
55. Cox CL, Payne-Johnson CE. Aural cholesterol granuloma in a dog. J Small Anim Pract 1995;36:25–8.
56. Fliegner RA, Jubb KV, Lording PM. Cholesterol granuloma associated with otitis media and destruction of the tympanic bulla in a dog. Vet Pathol 2007;44:547–9.
57. Hardie EM, Linder KE, Pease AP. Aural cholesteatoma in twenty dogs. Vet Surg 2008;37:763–70.
58. Greci V, Travetti O, Di Giancamillo M, et al. Middle ear cholesteatoma in 11 dogs. Can Vet J 2011;52:631–6.
59. Pratschke KM. Inflammatory polyps of the middle ear in 5 dogs. Vet Surg 2003; 32:292–6.
60. Blutke A, Parzefall B, Steger A, et al. Inflammatory polyp in the middle ear of a dog: a case report. Vet Med 2010;55:289–93.
61. Banco B, Grieco V, Di Giancamillo M, et al. Canine aural cholesteatoma: a histological and immunohistochemicalstudy. Vet J 2014;200:440–5.
62. Doust R, King A, Hammond G, et al. Assessment of middle ear disease in the dog: a comparison of diagnostic imaging modalities. J Small Anim Pract 2007; 48:188–92.
63. Travetti O, Giudice C, Greci V, et al. Computed tomography features of middle ear cholesteatoma in dogs. Vet Radiol Ultrasound 2010;51:374–9.
64. Foster A, Morandi F, May E. Prevalence of ear disease in dogs undergoing multidetector thin-slice computed tomography of the head. Vet Radiol Ultrasound 2015;56:18–24.
65. Newman AW, Estey CM, McDonough S, et al. Cholesteatoma and meningoencephalitis in a dog with chronic otitis externa. Vet Clin Pathol 2015;44:157–63.
66. Harran NX, Bradley KJ, Hetzel N, et al. MRI findings of a middle ear cholesteatoma in a dog. J Am Anim Hosp Assoc 2012;48:339–43.
67. Witsil AJ, Archipow W, Bettencourt AE, et al. What is your diagnosis? Cholesteatoma in a dog. J Am Vet Med Assoc 2013;243:775–7.
68. Leroith T, Binder EM, Graham AH, et al. Respiratory epithelial adenomatoid hamartoma in a dog. J Vet Diagn Invest 2009;21:918–20.
69. Osaki T, Takagi S, Hoshino Y, et al. Temporary regression of locally invasive polypoid rhinosinusitis in a dog after photodynamic therapy. Aust Vet J 2012; 90:442–7.
70. Holt DE, Goldschmidt MH. Nasal polyps in dogs: five cases (2005 to 2011). J Small Anim Pract 2011;52:660–3.
71. LaDouceur EE, Michel AO, Lindl Bylicki BJ, et al. Nasal cavity masses resembling chondro-osseous respiratory epithelial adenomatoid hamartomas in 3 dogs. Vet Pathol 2015;52. [Epub ahead of print].
72. Weinreb I. Low grade glandular lesions of the sinonasal tract: a focused review. Head Neck Pathol 2010;4:77–83.
73. Khan RA, Chernock RD, Lewis JS Jr. Seromucinous hamartoma of the nasal cavity: a report of two cases and review of the literature. Head Neck Pathol 2011;5: 241–7.
74. Fedda F, Boulos F, Sabri A. Chondro-osseous respiratory epithelial adenomatoid hamartoma of the nasal cavity. Int Arch Otorhinolaryngol 2013;17:218–21.
75. Li Y, Yang QX, Tian XT, et al. Malignant transformation of nasal chondromesenchymal hamartoma in adult: a case report and review of the literature. Histol Histopathol 2013;28:337–44.

Reconstruction of Congenital Nose, Cleft Primary Palate, and Lip Disorders

CrossMark

Nadine Fiani, BVSc[a], Frank J.M. Verstraete, DrMedVet, MMedVet[b], Boaz Arzi, DVM[b],*

KEYWORDS

- Cleft surgery • Cleft palate • Primary palate • Cleft lip

KEY POINTS

- Embryologic formation of the primary and secondary palates is important to the understanding of cleft palate development.
- Etiology of cleft formation has been described in the human literature but is lacking in the veterinary field.
- A clinical approach to the repair of the cleft of the primary palate includes: diagnostic tests, surgical repair of various configurations of the cleft, postoperative care, potential complications, and outcome.
- Surgical repair of clefts of the primary palate can be challenging; a thorough understanding of the anatomy in the region as well as important surgical principles must be adhered to for best outcome.

 Video content accompanies this article at http://www.vetsmall.theclinics.com

Clefts of the primary palate in the dog are uncommon, and their repair can be challenging.[1] The aims of this article are to provide information regarding pathogenesis and convey practical information for the repair of these defects.

EMBRYOLOGIC FORMATION OF THE PALATE

It is helpful to understand that, during embryogenesis, the separation between the nasal and oral cavities is formed in 2 stages, namely the primary and secondary palates:

Primary Palate

The primary palate forms first. It consists of the upper lip and incisive bones rostral to the palatine fissures.[2-5] The paired maxillary processes grow medially and push the

The authors have nothing to disclose.
[a] Department of Clinical Sciences, College of Veterinary Medicine, Cornell University, 602 Tower Road, Ithaca, NY 14853, USA; [b] Department of Surgical and Radiological Sciences, School of Veterinary Medicine, University of California - Davis, 1 Garrod Drive, Davis, CA 95616, USA
* Corresponding author.
E-mail address: barzi@ucdavis.edu

Vet Clin Small Anim 46 (2016) 663–675
http://dx.doi.org/10.1016/j.cvsm.2016.02.001
0195-5616/16/$ – see front matter © 2016 Elsevier Inc. All rights reserved.
vetsmall.theclinics.com

medial and lateral nasal processes toward the midline, where they all merge to form the base of the nose and the upper lip.[2,3] The 2 medial processes eventually form the incisive bone rostral to the palatine fissures.[2]

Secondary Palate

The secondary palate consists of the hard palate caudal to the palatine fissures and the soft palate. Following the formation of the primary palate, 3 outgrowths appear in the primitive oral cavity. The vomer grows ventrally from the frontonasal process along the midline, and the left and right palatine processes grow horizontally from the maxillary processes toward midline. The vomer and palatine processes fuse together at the midline and rostrally with the incisive bone, separating the oral and nasal cavities.[2,3,5]

PALATAL CLEFTS

Cleft lip (CL) is a term used to describe a fissure involving the structures of the primary palate.[3,4] The terms cleft lip and cleft of the primary palate are often used synonymously in the veterinary and human literature; however, neither is specific.[5,6] They could refer to a variety of combinations and severity of defects.[4,7] An incomplete CL may only present as a notch in the lip or reach part of the way toward, but not into, the nostril. A complete cleft will include all of the lip and continue into the nostril. A complete cleft is usually, but not always, accompanied by a cleft of the alveolar process and the incisive bone rostral to the palatine fissures. The extent of incisive bone involvement may also vary. CL defects may be unilateral or bilateral.

Cleft palate (CP) is a fissure involving the structures of the secondary palate. The severity of these clefts may vary from a small notch in the caudal aspect of the soft palate to a through-and-through defect involving the hard palate caudal to the palatine fissures and the entire soft palate.[4]

Historically, clefts have been divided into CL with or without CP (CL +/− CP) or CP only, as it has often been suggested that they are etiologically different (**Fig. 1**).[4,8,9] Clefts can further be classified as syndromic or nonsyndromic, whereby other physical or developmental anomalies are either present or absent, respectively.[6–8,10]

ETIOLOGY

The precise etiology of congenital clefts is unknown; however, genetic and environmental factors (ie, multifactorial etiology) are known to be involved.[11]

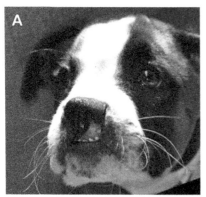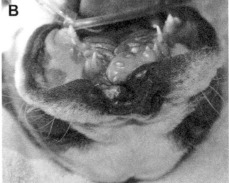

Fig. 1. (*A*) Exterior appearance of a puppy with a unilateral cleft lip. (*B*) Intraoral view of a puppy with a unilateral cleft of the primary palate and cleft of the secondary palate (CL + CP).

Genetic Factors

It is generally accepted that genetic factors play a leading role in the formation of facial clefts.[5] The incidence of CL +/− CP has been thoroughly documented in different ethnic groups, as well as familial recurrence in humans.[7,8,12,13] Most of the available veterinary studies identify affected puppies within relatively small, purebred and often inbred groups.[14–19] These findings provide strong evidence for genetic differences in susceptibility. Regions of several chromosomes have been identified as the candidates for the genes contributing to CL +/− CP.[20–22] Several specific genes that alter signaling molecules, transcription factors, or growth hormones in the developing face, have been identified.[5,7] Errors in any of those mechanisms can result in cleft formation.

Environmental Teratogens

Teratogens are substances capable of interfering with the development of a fetus and causing birth defects including facial and oral clefts.[23] Several chemicals and pharmaceutical agents including folic acid, aspirin, and certain antiepileptic drugs have been identified as playing a role in the formation of CL +/− CP.[5,24–27] Teratogens are thought to act on susceptible genotypes to produce the malformation, which may account in a large part for the individual variability in outcomes despite a similar degree of exposure.[23,24] Stage of gestation at the time of exposure to a teratogen has also been shown to be of great importance in the formation of CL +/− CP.[28,29]

CLEFTS OF THE PRIMARY PALATE IN THE VETERINARY LITERATURE

The number of veterinary studies and case reports referring to this topic is small.[9,15–17,19,30] Given the lack of large-scale studies and the great variations in phenotypic descriptions along with the frequent lack of diagnostic imaging, it is difficult to draw any major conclusions regarding breed predisposition, phenotypic appearance or other, possibly subtle, systemic abnormalities. However, with advanced genetic analysis and imaging technology, characterization of these clefts is becoming more common.

CLINICAL APPROACH TO DOGS WITH CLEFT OF THE PRIMARY PALATE

Although clefts of the primary plate can occur along with clefts of the secondary palate, the discussion will be limited only to reconstruction of clefts of the primary palate.

Diagnosis and Clinical Signs

Clefts of the primary palate involving the lip are obvious at birth.[29] Although these clefts render a puppy overtly abnormal in appearance, they are not commonly associated with acutely significant or life-threatening disease.[27] Puppies with wider clefts, especially those involving the floor of the nose and incisive bone, resulting in a communication between the nasal and oral cavities, may present with signs related to rhinitis. This is especially true when they start to eat on their own.[1,10] In severe cases, aspiration pneumonia may occur.

Necessity for Surgical Intervention

Clefts involving the lip alone are largely aesthetic and many do not require surgical treatment. However, clefts involving the nasal floor, alveolar margin, and incisive bone should be repaired. Although patients with the latter defect may not show overt clinical signs early in life, over time, food and other debris will become lodged in the defect. This will lead to inflammation of the nasal mucosa and eventual chronic rhinitis.

Age at the Time of Intervention

The age of the puppy at the time of intervention is of vital importance for 2 reasons, namely maxillofacial growth and dental development.[1]

Surgical manipulation of the palatal mucoperiosteum in puppies has been shown to interfere with and retard maxillary growth.[31,32] Periosteal elevation to create the mucogingival flaps necessary for the repair of clefts of the incisive bone is often needed. Proceeding with this at an early age may lead to abnormal facial growth or even dehiscence of the surgical site. If the puppy is not overly symptomatic, waiting until maxillofacial growth has slowed or even ceased completely prior to definitive surgery is preferred.[29]

Clefts of the primary palate often involve the alveolar margin and therefore the dental arch. It may be tempting to address the defect while the puppy still has deciduous dentition, as these teeth are small, and therefore relatively more soft tissue is available for repair. However, it must be noted that the permanent teeth, when they erupt, may interfere with the repair or may be forced to erupt into an abnormal position.[1] It is ideal to wait until the puppy's permanent incisor and canine teeth have completed their eruption (ie, 4–6 months) prior to considering surgical treatment.

Diagnostic Imaging

Diagnostic imaging plays an important role in surgical planning and must be performed prior to attempting repair.[10] The gold standard imaging modality of the head is computed tomography (CT).[33] This allows the reconstruction of 3-dimensional images of the bone defect and the surrounding dentition and informs the surgeon on the availability of bone support prior to surgical correction. It has been shown that the CP bone defect is often larger than the soft tissue defect.[10] Bone plays an important role in terms of surgical repair, as it acts as a scaffold, offering support for soft tissue flaps positioned over it.[1] Understanding the size of the bone defect and the location of surrounding dentition helps with surgical planning and gives an indication of prognosis. CT imaging can also provide information regarding the nasal cavity and especially the degree of nasal turbinate destruction.

Dental radiographs are important in the evaluation of the dentition adjacent to the defect or those involved directly within the defect. Malformed teeth or teeth that are present in an abnormal position and require extractions prior to surgical correction of the cleft are best assessed by dental radiography prior to extractions. Both CT and dental radiographs should ideally be used as part of the surgical planning.

Systemic Considerations

A thorough general physical examination, including thoracic auscultation, is always indicated prior to considering surgical treatment. If aspiration pneumonia is suspected, 3-view thoracic radiographs are indicated. It is important to treat and resolve the aspiration pneumonia prior to embarking on surgical intervention to correct the cleft lip and primary palate.

Complete blood count, biochemistry panel, and urinalysis should also be performed as part of the complete preanesthetic assessment.

Principles of Surgical Repair

The main objective of the surgical repair of clefts of the primary palate is to create a separation between the oral and nasal cavities.[1,29] Although the lip is the most obvious defect, its repair in the dog is largely aesthetic and is of secondary importance to the repair of the cleft of the incisive bone and floor of the nose.[29]

Repair of the primary palate is an invasive procedure, and regional nerve blocks need to be considered as a means of decreasing nociceptive input into the central nervous system (CNS) and therefore providing preemptive analgesia.[34] Bilateral infraorbital nerve blocks using a local anesthetic, such as bupivacaine, administered 10 to 15 minutes prior to commencing surgery, is recommended.

Preoperative antibiotics are indicated in the case of major oral surgery, such as cleft repair.[35] Ampicillin at 20 mg/kg administered intravenously 20 minutes prior to the commencement of surgery is the current antibiotic of choice. If the surgery is prolonged, a second dose should be administered after 6 hours.

The labial skin is clipped, and a preliminary scrub is performed. The patient is then positioned in dorsal recumbency; a pharyngeal pack is placed, and the oral cavity is irrigated with 0.12% chlorhexidine gluconate. All of the teeth are ultrasonically scaled supra and subgingivally. The mouth is then thoroughly flushed and suctioned. The nasal cavity should also be carefully suctioned to remove any debris and mucous. The labial skin and nasal planum are surgically prepared.

Although several texts advise repairing clefts of the primary palate with the patient in sternal recumbency,[1,29] the authors find that placing the patient in dorsal recumbency, at least initially, allows for improved access to the oral cavity and reconstruction of the nasal floor. Gravity naturally retracts the lips, improving visualization of the incisive bone, alveolar margin, and mucosa. Sterile drapes are applied to isolate the oral cavity and nasal planum.

Dental Implications: Strategic Extractions and Staged Repair

As discussed previously, it is best to allow the rostral maxillary permanent dentition to complete its eruption prior to definitive surgical repair. Strategic dental extractions may be necessary for one of the following reasons:

There is minimal soft tissue, and extraction will allow for more tissue to be harvested for definitive treatment.

The teeth are erupting directly into the cleft and will greatly interfere with soft tissue closure.

In cases in which minimal tissue is available, a staged approach is preferred. Diagnostic imaging is performed and studied to help design a plan for strategic extraction of some or all maxillary incisor teeth plus or minus canine teeth under the first anesthetic event. The extraction sites are allowed to heal for approximately 4 to 6 weeks before definitive cleft repair is considered.

In some cases, if incisor teeth are growing directly into the cleft, simple extraction of the offending teeth at the time of definitive repair may be adequate.

REPAIR OF THE UNILATERAL CLEFT OF THE PRIMARY PALATE

Clefts of the primary palate are repaired in three steps, which are also described in **Fig. 2**:

Repair of the Palatal Defect

A No. 15 scalpel blade is used to create a full-thickness mucoperiosteal pedicle flap at the rostral aspect of the palate, lateral to the defect (see **Fig. 2**D). The flap extends from the level of the first or second premolar tooth to the canine tooth and connects with a tangential incision made at the edge of the bone defect. The incision may be extended along the midline of the palate if needed. Care should be taken when incising mucosa close to the gingiva so as not to disrupt the sulcular anatomy. A periosteal

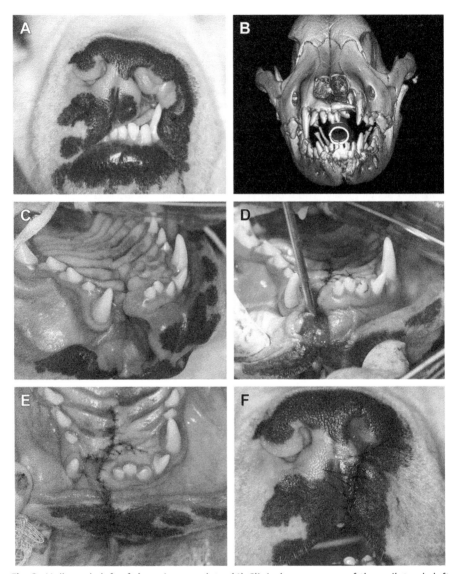

Fig. 2. Unilateral cleft of the primary palate. (*A*) Clinical appearance of the unilateral cleft extraorally. (*B*) CT reconstruction demonstrating the rostral aspect of the cleft. Note the left maxillary second and third incisor teeth growing toward the defect. (*C*) Intraoral image showing unilateral cleft. The maxillary second and third incisors had been extracted approximately 4 weeks prior (at the time the CT was obtained). (*D*) Palatal pedicle flap relocated medially and sutured over the defect. Instrument pointing to apposed orbicularis oris muscle and nasal mucosa. (*E*) Complete reconstruction of the intraoral defect. (*F*) Extraoral reconstructed lip and nasal floor.

elevator is then used to elevate the pedicle and mobilize it medially toward the incisive bone and over the cleft.

The oral mucosa covering the edge of the incisive bone is also tangentially incised and elevated to help form a shelf for suturing. It is not usually necessary to mobilize the incisive tissues. If possible, the nasal mucosa should be elevated on either side of the defect and apposed first using 4-0 or 5-0 poliglecaprone 25 on a cutting needle in a simple-interrupted pattern with the knots facing the oral cavity. This is only possible if the cleft is narrow, as the nasal tissue cannot be easily mobilized toward the midline of the cleft. The pedicle flap can then be repositioned toward the incisive bone, and the edges of the oral mucosa can be apposed using 4-0 or 5-0 poliglecaprone 25 in a simple-interrupted pattern.

Repair of the Floor of the Nose, Gingival Margin, Alveolar Mucosa, and Labial Mucosa

A No. 11 scalpel blade is used to make a tangential incision along the gingival margin, alveolar mucosa and buccal mucosa on either side of the cleft (see **Fig. 2**D and E). A periosteal elevator is used to elevate the nasal mucosa on either side of the alveolar margin defect. The nasal mucosa deep to the gingival and alveolar margins should be apposed in a simple-interrupted pattern. This will recreate the floor of the nose. The orbicularis oris muscle should be closed next, allowing for the start of the labial reconstruction. The oral mucosa, consisting of gingiva, alveolar mucosa, and labial mucosa, can be directly apposed in cases where the cleft is narrow. However, if the cleft is wide and there is tension at the site of apposition, further flap design may be necessary. A commonly used method is to create a pedicle flap using the alveolar mucosa on 1 side to the defect. The flap is carefully undermined using Metzenbaum scissors. The pedicle flap is advanced caudally so that it is bound by gingiva on the lateral and medial aspects and palatal mucosa at its most apical point.

Repair of the Lip, Nasal Planum, and the Rostral Portion of the Floor of the Nose

This final part of the repair is most practically performed with the patient in sternal recumbency (see **Fig. 2**F). A tangential incision of the mucocutaneous junctions has already been performed as part of the intraoral repair. The incision, however, must be extended dorsally into the nasal planum and floor of the nose. The labial skin, nasal planum, and floor of the nose on either side of the cleft are directly apposed in a simple-interrupted pattern (Video 1). If there is tension at the surgical site at the time of closure, several techniques have been described in the human literature to alleviate this.[4] Some of these techniques have been adapted to the canine patient.[1,29]

REPAIR OF BILATERAL CLEFT OF THE PRIMARY PALATE

In the case of bilateral clefts, the previously described 3 steps are performed; however, they are done bilaterally (**Fig. 3**). Care must be taken with the repair of the lip and nasal planum as there may be tensions across the skin repair. Further mobilization of the skin may be necessary. It is common for the lip to appear short or give a notched appearance following bilateral repair. If there is no tension at the surgical site, this is not considered a clinical problem.

REPAIR OF SEVERE BILATERAL CLEFT OF THE PRIMARY PALATE—SALVAGE INCISIVECTOMY

In cases of extensive bilateral clefts, reconstruction may not be possible due to the lack of soft tissue or due to great instability of the incisive bones. In these cases, an incisivectomy may be the best option to allow for successful repair and maximum function (**Fig. 4**).

The patient is prepared as described previously, and placed in dorsal recumbency. A No. 11 scalpel blade is used to perform tangential incisions on the lateral aspect of the incisive bone. These incisions are then made continuous with sulcular incisions

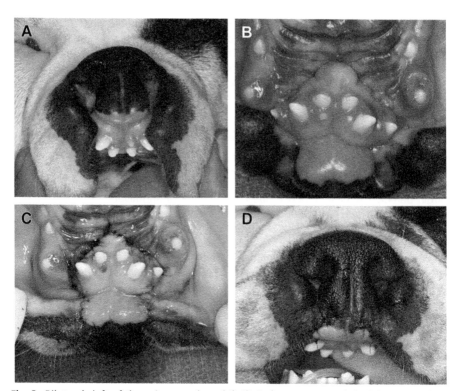

Fig. 3. Bilateral cleft of the primary palate. (*A*) Clinical appearance of the bilateral cleft extraorally. (*B*) Intraoral appearance. (*C*) Intraoral repair. (*D*) Extraoral reconstruction of lip and nasal floor.

around all the incisors within the incisive bones (see **Fig. 4**C). A periosteal elevator is used to elevate the nasal mucosa on the lateral aspects of the incisive bones along with the alveolar mucosa on the labial aspect (see **Fig. 4**D). This will result in exposure of the incisive bones and the incisor teeth and will make soft tissues more available for reconstruction and closure. A bone-cutting instrument is then used to transect the vomer and remove the incisive bones.

Once the incisive bone is removed, tangential incisions are made along the edges of the palate. A periosteal elevator is used to elevate and reflect the nasal mucosa dorsally and the palatal mucosa ventrally. The nasal mucosa is apposed. The gingiva and alveolar mucosa that were elevated from the incisive bone is advanced caudally so that its edges can be sutured to the palatal mucosa, therefore closing the palatal defect bilaterally (see **Fig. 4**E). The alveolar and labial mucosa on either side of the defects is also directly apposed in 2 simple-interrupted layers, therefore recreating the nasal floor along with the oral vestibule respectively. Using a simple-interrupted pattern allows good opposition and helps to avoid inversion of the tissues. The patient is then placed in sternal recumbency, and reconstruction of the labial skin and nasal planum is performed as described previously (see **Fig. 4**F).

REPAIR OF THE BIFID NOSE—CENTRAL CLEFT

The bifid nose is an extremely rare midline facial cleft, with only 1 report available in the veterinary literature (**Fig. 5**).[30] A brief explanation of the technique is provided here.

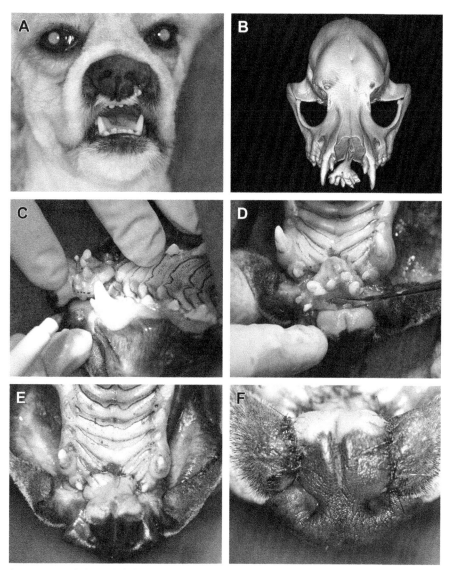

Fig. 4. Severe bilateral clef to the primary palate. (*A*) Clinical appearance of the bilateral cleft extraorally. (*B*) CT reconstruction showing severity and bony extent of the bilateral defects. (*C*) Surgical marker used to demarcate incision line with the aim of retaining as much soft tissue as possible. (*D*) Periosteal elevator used to elevate the soft tissues away from the incisive bone. (*E*) Palatal repair once the incisive bone is removed. (*F*) Extraoral of reconstructed lip and nasal floor.

With the dog in sternal recumbency, the surgical margins are outlined, and stay sutures are placed at the outlined margins. A Y-shaped skin incision is made over the dorsal midline of the nasal bones with the widest portion on the excision at the bifid philtrum area. The incision is extended to the subcutaneous and cartilaginous tissue. Following removal of the central portion of the skin and subcutaneous tissue, the

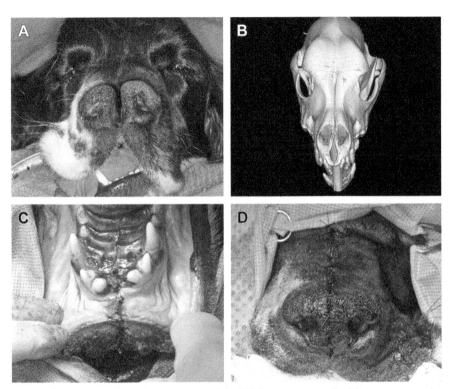

Fig. 5. Bifid nose. (*A*) Clinical appearance of the bifid nose extraorally. (*B*) CT reconstruction of the defect. (*C*) Reconstruction of the intraoral defect. (*D*) Extraoral reconstruction of the lip, nasal planum, and dorsal aspect of the nose.

cartilaginous septum is brought to the midline (which in the normal state is unpaired). The dorsal lateral nasal cartilages and the nasal cartilaginous septum are reapposed to the correct anatomic position and sutured. The subcutaneous tissues, skin, and nasal planum are then apposed directly and sutured. The dog is then repositioned into dorsal recumbency. The intraoral approach to the cleft is performed as previously described in this article.

POSTOPERATIVE CARE AND COMPLICATIONS
Postoperative Care

In the immediate postoperative phase, the patient must be hospitalized and administered intravenous or subcutaneous analgesic medications. The authors' preference is to administer a nonsteroidal anti-inflammatory (NSAID) on recovery along with a continuous-rate infusion of fentanyl at 3 to 5 μg/kg/h. The following day, if the patient is eating, it is given an oral NSAID and Tramadol for 7 days.

The patient is administered ampicillin intravenously every 6 hours for the following 12 hours. The morning following surgery, the patient should be given oral amoxicillin and clavulanic acid, 15 to 20 mg/kg every 12 hours for 7 days.

The patient is hand-fed soft or canned food once fully conscious following anesthesia. Hand feeding small portions regularly (every 8 hours) is recommended for the first 24 to 48 hours after surgery. After that point, patients can eat comfortably from a bowl on their own. The dog should be continued on the soft for 3 weeks following surgery. If the surgical site appears to have healed well, the patient can then return to a normal diet including hard food.

An Elizabethan collar is applied prior to recovery to prevent any self-inflicting trauma. It should be kept on at all times for 2 weeks.

The client must be made aware of the danger of wound dehiscence if the dog chews on a hard object. All access to these must be strictly prohibited for 3 weeks.

If the dog is eating and taking oral medications well, it can be sent home the day following its surgical repair. The authors recommend rechecking the patient at 2 weeks to assess healing and then again at 4 weeks to assess overall appearance and function.

Complications

Wound dehiscence is the most common complication. The most frequent causes for this are tension at the surgical site and poor surgical technique. If wound breakdown does occur, it is best to let the tissues heal by second intention and to attempt a second repair once the soft tissues have healed and are no longer inflamed and friable. It is important to realize, however, that numerous attempts at surgical repair may be more difficult due to fibrous scar formation and soft tissue contracture. Another possible cause for dehiscence is occlusal trauma caused by the mandibular canine tooth. It is prudent to assess dental occlusion immediately after cleft repair. If the mandibular canine tooth is occluding into the surgical site, crown height reduction and vital pulp therapy or extraction should be considered.

SUMMARY

Clefts of the primary palate are not well described or characterized in the veterinary literature, and no accurate or practical classification system yet exists. Surgical repair of the clefts of the primary palate can be challenging. A thorough understanding of the anatomy in the region as well as important surgical principles must be adhered to for best results.

SUPPLEMENTARY DATA

Supplementary data related to this article can be found at http://dx.doi.org/10.1016/j.cvsm.2016.02.001.

REFERENCES

1. Manfra SM. Cleft palate repair techniques. In: Verstraete FJM, Lommer MJ, editors. Oral and maxillofacial surgery in dogs and cats. Edinburgh (United Kingdom): Saunders Elsevier; 2012. p. 351–61.

2. Nanci A. Embryology of the head, face and oral cavity. In: Dolan J, editor. Ten cate's oral hisology development, structure and function. 7th edition. St Louis (MO): Mosby Elsevier; 2008. p. 32–56.

3. James JN, Costello BJ, Ruiz RL. Management of cleft lip and palate and cleft orthognathic considerations. Oral Maxillofac Surg Clin North Am 2014;26(4): 565–72.

4. Ellis E. Management of patients with orofacial clefts. In: Hupp JR, editor. Contemporary oral and maxillofacial surgery. 5th edition. St Louis (MO): Mosby Elsevier; 2008. p. 583–603.

5. Kelly KM, Bardach J. Biologic basis of cleft palate and palatal surgery. In: Verstraete FJM, Lommer MJ, editors. Oral and maxillofacial surgery in dogs and cats. Edinburgh (United Kingdom): Saunders Elsevier; 2012. p. 343–50.

6. Wang KH, Heike CL, Clarkson MD, et al. Evaluation and integration of disparate classification systems for clefts of the lip. Front Physiol 2014;5:1–11.

7. Bender PL. Genetics of cleft lip and palate. J Pediatr Nurs 2000;15(4):242–9.

8. Dixon MJ, Marazita ML, Beaty TH, et al. Cleft lip and palate: understanding genetic and environmental influences. Nat Rev Genet 2011;12(3):167–78.

9. Dreyer CJ, Preston CB. Classification of cleft lip and palate in animals. Cleft Palate J 1974;11:327–32.

10. Nemec A, Daniaux L, Jonson E, et al. Craniomaxillofacial abnormalities in dogs with congenital palatal defects: computed tomographic findings. Vet Surg 2015;44:417–22.

11. Meng L, Bian Z, Torensma R, et al. Biological mechanisms in palatogenesis and cleft palate. J Dent Res 2009;88(1):22–33.

12. Nouri N, Memarzadeh M, Carinci F, et al. Family-based association analysis between nonsyndromic cleft lip with or without cleft palate and IRF6 polymorphism in an Iranian population. Clin Oral Investig 2015;19(4):891–4.

13. Mostowska A, Hozyasz KK, Wójcicki P, et al. Association between polymorphisms at the GREM1 locus and the risk of nonsyndromic cleft lip with or without cleft palate in the Polish population. Birth Defects Res A Clin Mol Teratol 2015;103(10): 847–56.

14. Senders CW, Eisele P, Freeman LE, et al. Observations about the normal and abnormal embryogenesis of the canine lip and palate. J Craniofac Genet Dev Biol Suppl 1986;2:241–8.

15. Natsume N, Miyajima K, Kinoshita H, et al. Incidence of cleft lip and palate in beagles. Plast Reconstr Surg 1994;93(2):439.

16. Richtsmeier JT, Sack GH, Grausz HM, et al. Cleft palate with autosomal recessive transmission in Brittany spaniels. Cleft Palate Craniofac J 1994;31(5):364–71.

17. Kemp C, Thiele H, Dankof A, et al. Cleft lip and/or palate with monogenic autosomal recessive transmission in pyrenees shepherd dogs. Cleft Palate Craniofac J 2009;46(1):81–8.

18. Moura E, Cirio SM, Pimpão CT. Nonsyndromic cleft lip and palate in boxer dogs: evidence of monogenic autosomal recessive inheritance. Cleft Palate Craniofac J 2012;49(6):759–60.

19. Wolf ZT, Brand HA, Shaffer JR, et al. Genome-wide association studies in dogs and humans identify ADAMTS20 as a risk variant for cleft lip and palate. PLoS Genet 2015;11(3):e1005059.

20. Wolf ZT, Leslie EJ, Arzi B, et al. A LINE-1 Insertion in DLX6is responsible for cleft palate and mandibular abnormalities in a canine model of Pierre Robin sequence. PLoS Genet 2014;10(4):e1004257.

21. Prabhu S, Krishnapillai R, Jose M, et al. Etiopathogenesis of orofacial clefting revisited. J Oral Maxillofac Pathol 2012;16(2):228–32.

22. Rajendran R, Shaikh SF, Anil S. Tracing disease gene(s) in non-syndromic clefts of orofacial region: HLA haplotypic linkage by analyzing the microsatellite markers: MIB, C1_2_5, C1_4_1, and C1_2_A. Indian J Hum Genet 2011;17(3): 188–93.

23. Young DL, Schneider RA, Hu D, et al. Genetic and teratogenic approaches to craniofacial development. Crit Rev Oral Biol Med 2000;11(3):304–17.

24. Inoyama K, Meador KJ. Cognitive outcomes of prenatal antiepileptic drug exposure. Epilepsy Res 2015;114:89–97.

25. Elwood JM, Colquhoun TA. Observations on the prevention of cleft palate in dogs by folic acid and potential relevance to humans. N Z Vet J 1997;45(6):254–6.
26. Robertson RT, Allen HL, Bokelman DL. Aspirin: teratogenic evaluation in the dog. Teratology 1979;20(2):313–20.
27. Jurkiewicz MJ, Bryant DL. Cleft lip and palate in dogs: a progress report. Cleft Palate J 1968;5:30–6.
28. Syska E, Schmidt R, Schubert J. The time of palatal fusion in mice: a factor of strain susceptibility to teratogens. J Craniomaxillofac Surg 2004;32(1):2–4.
29. Nelson AW. Cleft palate. In: Slatter DH, editor. Textbook of small animal surgery, vol. 1, 3rd edition. Philadelphia: Saunders Elsevier; 2003. p. 814–23.
30. Arzi B, Verstraete FJM. Repair of a bifid nose combined with a cleft of the primary palate in a 1-year-old dog. Vet Surg 2011;40(7):865–9.
31. Kremenak CR, Huffman WC, Olin WH. Growth of maxillae in dogs after palatal surgery I. Cleft Palate J 1970;4:6–17.
32. Kremenak CR, Huffman WC, Olin WH. Growth of maxillae in dogs after palatal surgery II. Cleft Palate J 1967;7:719–36.
33. Bar-Am Y, Pollard RE, Kass PH, et al. The diagnostic yield of conventional radiographs and computed tomography in dogs and cats with maxillofacial trauma. Vet Surg 2008;37(3):294–9.
34. Pascoe PJ. Anesthesia and pain management. In: Verstraete FJM, Lommer MJ, editors. Oral and maxillofacial surgery in dogs and cats. Edinburgh (United Kingdom): Saunders Elsevier; 2012. p. 23–42.
35. Sarkiala-Kessel EM. Use of antibiotics and antiseptics. In: Verstraete FJM, Lommer MJ, editors. Oral and maxillofacial surgery in dogs and cats. Edinburgh (United Kingdom): Saunders Elsevier; 2012. p. 15–21.

Diagnosis and Management of Nasopharyngeal Stenosis

Allyson C. Berent, DVM

KEYWORDS

- Nasopharyngeal stenosis • Choanal atresia • Balloon dilation
- Nasopharyngeal stenting • Covered metallic stent
- Balloon expandable metallic stent • Self-expanding metallic stent

KEY POINTS

- Choanal atresia is rare in small animal veterinary medicine, and most cases are misdiagnosed and are actually a nasopharyngeal stenosis.
- Nasopharyngeal stenosis is a frustrating disease to treat because of the high recurrence rates encountered after surgical intervention.
- Minimally invasive treatment options like balloon dilation (BD), metallic stent placement (MS), or covered metallic stent (CMS) placement have been met with good success but are associated with various complications that must be considered.
- The most common complication with BD alone is stenosis recurrence in over 70% of cases.
- The most common complications encountered with MS placement is tissue in-growth, chronic infections and the development of an oronasal fistula. The most common complications with a CMS is chronic infections and the development of an oronasal fistula, but stricture recurrence is avoided.

Nasopharyngeal stenosis (NPS) is a pathologic narrowing within the nasopharynx, which is the cavity caudal to the choanae above the hard and soft palate. This condition results in inspiratory and expiratory stertor that is static, especially during breathing when the mouth is closed. This can occur as a congenital anomaly similar to choanal atresia, or, more commonly, secondary to an inflammatory condition like chronic rhinitis, aspiration rhinitis, surgical manipulation, trauma, or a tumor/polyp.[1–7] The most common reason NPS is seen in dogs is due to aspiration rhinitis after an anesthesia event,[4,6,8,9] and in cats, it is most often found at the time of a rescue situation, suspected to be caused by chronic inflammatory disease, herpes virus, or congenital scar tissue development.[10] Nasopharyngeal stenosis has only been described in the veterinary literature in a small number of cases,[1–9,11–13] and it

Department of Interventional Radiology and Endoscopy, Internal Medicine, The Animal Medical Center, 510 East 62nd Street, New York, NY 10065, USA
E-mail address: Allyson.Berent@amcny.org

Vet Clin Small Anim 46 (2016) 677–689
http://dx.doi.org/10.1016/j.cvsm.2016.01.005
0195-5616/16/$ – see front matter © 2016 Elsevier Inc. All rights reserved.

vetsmall.theclinics.com

was recently reported in abstract form in 46 dogs and cats.[10] Minimally invasive interventions are typically recommended due to the high rate of recurrence after palatal surgeries.[1–14] The most common approaches have been balloon dilation,[6–12] metallic stent placement,[3,6,9,10] or a temporary silicone tubing after stenosis dilation.[15] All have been shown to be effective for various indications but can be associated with recurrence and various complications.[1–15]

CLINICAL PRESENTATION

Respiratory signs are often consistent with a fixed obstruction that is both inspiratory and expiratory in nature, and resolves with open mouth breathing. Animals can be severely stertorous, dyspneic, or mildly noisy; they can have chronic regurgitation caused by an associated sliding hiatal hernia and megaesophagus. Additionally, they can be obligate open mouth breathers or can have chronic nasal discharge, experience gagging and repeated swallowing, chronic upper respiratory infections, chronic otitis media, and sneezing.[1–15] A thorough history of chronic upper respiratory infections, recent anesthetic events, otitis, or prior surgery is very important.

DIAGNOSIS

The diagnosis of nasopharyngeal stenosis is made during retroflex rhinoscopy of the nasopharynx using a flexible endoscope (**Fig. 1**). Computed tomography (CT) can also be diagnostic, but if the slices are too large, this lesion can be missed (**Fig. 2**). The author typically recommends 1 mm slices, which help identify the lesion and get an exact measurement of the stenosis length and nasopharyngeal diameter, both rostral and caudal to the stenosis (see **Fig. 2**). Imaging should be done from the tip of the nares to the larynx, including the entire nose and nasopharynx, as many patients have concurrent chronic rhinitis. It is also important to realize that most of these patients have an accumulation of mucous rostral to this lesion, and this is often misdiagnosed on CT as a longer stenosis than is actually present. This makes definitive characterization of the lesion length more accurate during retroflex rhinoscopy and antegrade contrast nasopharyngoscopy (**Fig. 3**) The tympanic bullae are often mucous filled as well because of the failure of Eustachian tube drainage, which is impeded chronically by the presence of an NPS. This is rarely of clinical significance.

A thorough oral examination should be performed to ensure there are no palatal defects. These are rare but can be seen, and this may change the therapeutic approach taken.

The nasopharyngeal stenosis is characterized as either a patent membrane, meaning there is a hole through the center of the obstructive lesion (see **Fig. 1**) or an

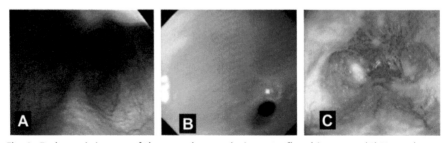

Fig. 1. Endoscopic images of the nasopharynx during retroflex rhinoscopy. (*A*) Normal nasopharynx in a dog. (*B*) Patent nasopharyngeal stenosis in a cat. (*C*) Imperforate nasopharyngeal stenosis in a dog.

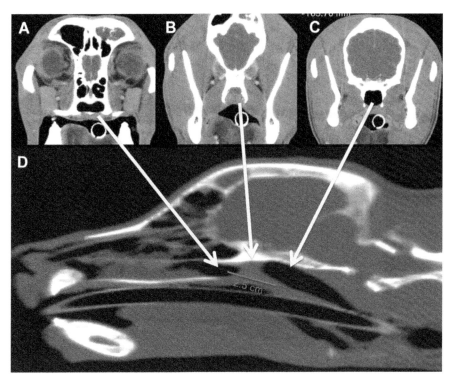

Fig. 2. CT images of a dog with NPS. (*A*) Transverse image of the nasopharynx rostral to the stenosis at the level of the hard palate. (*B*) Transverse image of the NPS at the stenosis. (*C*) Transverse image of the nasopharynx just caudal to the stenosis. (*D*) Sagittal image of the head showing the length of the nasopharyngeal stenosis in the rostral aspect of the nasopharynx measuring 2.5 cm long.

imperforate membrane, where the entire nasopharynx is closed from the stenotoic lesion (see **Fig. 1**). The imperforate membrane is more commonly seen in dogs than it is in cats, and it is most often associated with aspiration rhinitis or trauma, in the author's experience. The reason this differentiation is important is that they are treated differently and have a different prognosis. Imperforate membranes often behave more aggressively and are harder to maintain patency.

In a recent study[10] evaluating 46 patients with NPS (15 dogs and 31 cats), the median age was 2.4 years (range, 0.25–16.5 years); the cause of the stenosis was unknown in 45% of cases (had signs since adoption) or was associated with chronic rhinitis in 17%, known aspiration rhinitis 17% (7 dogs, 1 cat), chronic upper respiratory infections (9%), congenital webbing (6.5%) and trauma/surgery (4%).[10] The morphology of the stenosis was considered patent in 76% of cases (47% of dogs; 90% of cats) and imperforate in 24% of cases (53% of dogs, and 10% of cats).[10] The location of the stenosis was seen in the proximal/rostral nasopharynx in 39% of cases (87% of dogs, 16% of cats); mid-nasopharynx in 11% of cases (6.7% of dogs, 13% of cats); and caudal nasopharynx in 48% of cases (0% of dogs, 71% of cats).[10]

CLINICAL MANAGEMENT

Reported treatment options for NPS includes surgical resection, laser ablation, metallic stent placement (MS), covered metallic stent placement (CMS), and temporary stent

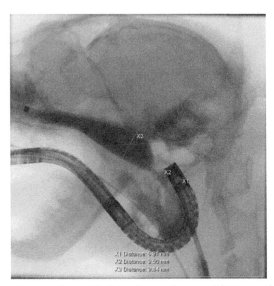

Fig. 3. Fluoroscopy images of a cat in lateral recumbency with a nasopharyngeal stenosis during a contrast nasopharyngeogram. Notice the marker catheter being used to measure the length of the stenosis and dorsoventral diameter of the nasopharynx.

placement (TS).[1–15] Various complications are associated with each option, and those will be highlighted (**Table 1**).

NPS can be in the rostral, mid or caudal nasopharynx, as mentioned previously. For lesions that are very thin (<5 mm) and are patent, balloon dilation alone is initially recommended, and seemingly more effective, in the author's experience. These lesions seem to have the highest chance of ultimate success, although in a recent report there was only 30% success after 1 balloon dilation.[10] For cats, where the lesions are typically thinner, patent, and in the caudal nasopharynx, the success rate with balloon dilation alone reaches 50%.[10]

PROCEDURE

The patient is placed in lateral recumbency, and a mouth gag is placed on the dependent canine teeth. Care should be taken to avoid overextension of the jaw. The anesthetist should be sure the endotracheal tube cuff is appropriately inflated, as contrast studies and rigorous flushing will occur and aspiration of fluid and contrast material should be avoided. In some cases, neuromuscular blockade is helpful to prevent excessive gagging during retroflex endoscope placement and other manipulations in this sensitive area.

The flexible bronchoscope should be placed in a retroflexed manner transorally and positioned over the soft palate into the nasopharynx so the NPS is clearly visualized (see **Fig. 3**). Under fluoroscopic guidance, a 0.035-inch hydrophilic angle-tipped guide wire is advanced through the naris, into the ventral nasal meatus, and directed caudally to the stenosis (see **Fig. 3**). For animals with patent NPS, the guide wire is directed through the small opening and down the esophagus.

For patients in which no orifice is visible a vascular access sheath (6–8 F) is advanced through the 1 naris, over the guide wire to the level of the stenosis (**Fig. 4**). To create an opening, the NPS is viewed via retroflexed rhinoscopy, and the scope is advanced rostrally to the stenosis to visualize the caudal aspect of the

Table 1
Complications associated with treatment of nasopharyngeal stenosis

	In-Growth	Chronic Infection	Fracture	ONF	Bending	Exag. Swallow	Migration	Removal	None
BD N = 27	70% after 1 treatment; 59% if > 1 treatment	NA	NA	NA	NA	NA	NA	NA	30% (11/22 cats; 0/5 dogs)
MS N = 30	33% (10)	23% (7)	17% (5)	13% (4)	6.7% (2)	6.7% (2)	6.7% (2)	3.3% (1)	30% (9)
CMS N = 11	0	54% (6)	0	27% (3)	0	0	9% (1)	9% (1)	36% (4)
Total N = 34	29% (10)	38% (13)	15% (5)	20% (7)	5.9% (2)	5.9% (2)	8.8% (3)	5.9% (2)	38% (13)

Abbreviations: BD, Balloon dilation; CMS, covered metallic stent placement; MS, metallic stent placement; ONF, oral–nasal fistula.

membrane. A guide wire can be used through the endoscope to mark the caudal aspect of the stenosis fluoroscopically (see **Fig. 4**). An 18 gauge renal access trocar needle is advanced through the access sheath to pierce the membrane, visualizing it simultaneously with rhinoscopy (see **Fig. 4**) and fluoroscopy. The needle is directed in a dorsomedial direction to avoid piercing the soft palate, and aiming to stay on midline. Once through the membrane, the stylette is removed, and the guide wire is advanced through the trocar needle and down the esophagus. The needle and sheath are removed, and an 8 Fr vascular dilator is passed over the wire to expand the orifice large enough to accept a balloon dilation catheter.

Next, the distal end of the stenosis is appreciated rhinoscopically and its location confirmed fluoroscopically using anatomic landmarks (ie, bullae or other landmarks) (see **Fig. 4**). An appropriately sized balloon dilation catheter that is strong enough to break this thick fibrous, or pseudocartilagenous, band (eg, 6–15 atmospheres of pressure rated burst pressure) is advanced over the guide wire, through the stenosis, and visualized endoscopically and fluoroscopically. The balloon is inflated with 50% iohexol and 50% saline solution via fluoroscopic guidance using an appropriate insufflation device (see **Fig. 4**). This should not be done with hand pressure, as it is typically not strong enough to efface the stricture. The waist of the stenosis is viewed to expand the stricture, and the balloon is deflated and removed over the wire. If no stent is being placed, then this balloon should be 1 mm larger than the predetermined diameter of the nasopharynx in this area. If a stent is to be placed, then the balloon diameter should be 50% to 60% of the nasopharyngeal diameter or the balloon-expandable metallic stent (BEMS) can just be placed primarily. It is important to remember that the animals with a totally closed imperforate stenosis are not typically ballooned alone as a sole procedure, as this has a high chance of recurrence (>95%).[10]

Balloon Dilation

This procedure is performed using both endoscopic and fluoroscopic guidance as described previously (see **Fig. 4**). Once the NPS is broken satisfactorily (see **Fig. 4**), topical 0.1% Mitomycin C can be instilled in the region of the stenosis. For cats, 2.5 mL are used, and for dogs, 5 mL are used. After 5 minutes, this region should be flushed vigorously with saline.[6] The operator and anesthetist should wear chemotherapy safety gloves during and after the infusion. Another alternative is endoscopic submucosal injections of 0.2 mg/kg of triamcinolone, divided into 4 quadrants.[6] This can be injected through the working channel of the bronchoscope using a flexible injection needle. Some operators advocate injecting the triamcinolone prior to effacing the stenosis and others after the mucosa is torn. It is important that the entire waist of the stenosis be seen to break under fluoroscopic guidance. If this is only done using endoscopic visualization, it is not uncommon to see mucosal tearing and assume that the stenosis is completely effaced. When the balloon dilation is done using a combination of both endoscopy and fluoroscopy you can appreciate when the true stenosis is broken as the waist on the balloon, under fluoroscopic visualization is also effaced.

The biggest complication with balloon dilation (BD) alone is the recurrence of the NPS. This usually occurs within 1 week to 1 month, but the author has seen recurrence at 6 to 12 months as well.[6,7,10] In a recent report[10] on 46 cases of NPS, 27 patients had BD performed initially. Of those 27 cases, 30% were successful in maintaining patency after 1 BD procedure, and 41% were successful after no more than 3 BD procedures. This success was seen in 50% of cats and 0% of dogs.[10] The cost of multiple procedures with the high rate of recurrence is what has forced investigation into the potential of more successful procedures.

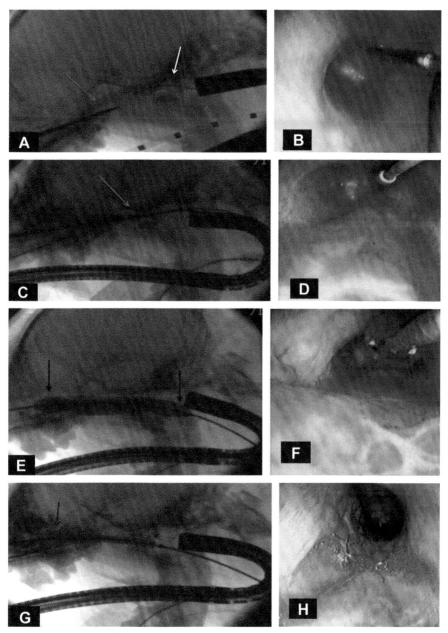

Fig. 4. Endoscopic and fluoroscopic images of an imperforate NPS during the piercing of the closed membrane. (*A*) Lateral fluoroscopic image during retroflex rhinoscopy showing the needle in the nasopharynx (*red arrow*) and a guide wire (*white arrow*) through the endoscope to mark the end of the stenosis. (*B*) Endoscopic image as the needle is passed through the stenosis. (*C*) Guide wire (*red arrow*) is passed through the needle creating a path for the balloon dilation to occur. (*D*) Same as seen in (*C*). (*E*) Balloon dilation (*black arrows*) of the imperforate stenosis using fluoroscopic and endoscopic (*F*) guidance. (*G*) Premounted nasopharyngeal stent (*Blue arrows*) passed over the guide wire under fluoroscopic guidance. (*H*) Endoscopic image after the stent is deployed showing a patent nasopharynx and the choanae at the rostral aspect of the cavity.

Nasopharyngeal Stenosis Metallic Stenting

When BD fails, or is declined as a first-line treatment option, then many clients consider nasopharyngeal stenting. This procedure is performed similar to that described previously for BD; only after the NPS is preballoon dilated (to about 50%–60% of the diameter predetermined based on either contrast study or CT), a stent is advanced over the wire, centered across the stenosis, and deployed using both endoscopic and fluoroscopic guidance (**Fig. 5**). There are different types of stents that can be used for this, either a BEMS or a self-expanding metallic stent (SEMS) (**Fig. 6**). Either of these stents can be covered (CMS-covered metallic stent) or uncovered (MS-metallic stent). For the BEMS, the balloon is inflated with a 50% contrast/50% saline mixture until the stenosis is effaced under fluoroscopic guidance (see **Fig. 5**). A SEMS is used if the stenosis is long (over 3 cm), when a covered stent is being considered (silicone-covered stents are usually SEMS types of stents), or if there is a history of BEMS compression. The SEMS is deployed differently than the BEMS. This stent is usually a woven metallic stent, similar to a tracheal stent. This stent is compressed down onto a delivery system, so it is actually longer on the delivery system than its ultimate length after deployment. This makes it much harder to predict the exact ultimate location and length once deployed, and more mistakes can be made if this stent is used without ample experience. Proper training is recommended prior to considering using these stents to understand the mechanisms of deployment.

If the stenosis is more caudally positioned within the nasopharynx, then it is important the operator leaves at least 1 cm of unstented soft palate caudal to the stent to prevent food from getting up into the nasopharynx. Similarly, if the stenosis is very rostral, just behind the choanae, care should be taken to know exactly where the nasal septum ends so the proximal end of the stent is not placed down 1 nasal passage. This will result in excessive mucous accumulation in the caged-off nasal passage, because drainage will be compromised. Sometimes this cannot be achieved, and the stent is placed on 1 side, especially in cases of choanal atresia; however, this is not ideal and should be avoided whenever possible. One way to help prevent this from occurring is to pass a red rubber catheter down each nasal passage so that one can endoscopically visualize through the predilated stenosis where the septum lies (where both catheters are seen to meet). This area is marked on the fluoroscopic image (using molars/hard palate location), or with the computed tomography (CT) scan, and the stent is then deployed caudal to this region. When choanal atresia occurs, 2 stents can be deployed in each nasal passage, where they meet in the nasopharynx. This is termed "kissing stents, or double barrel." Choanal atresia is extremely rare in dogs and cats, so this approach is not typically necessary, despite the common misdiagnosis for NPS. Most diagnosed choanal atresia cases are actually NPS once they are investigated more carefully.

Following stent deployment, delivery system is removed over the wire, leaving the expanded stent in place across the now-expanded lesion (see **Fig. 5**). A catheter is placed over the wire; the wire is removed, and vigorous nasal flushing is performed with sterile saline solution to try and clear the nasal passages and sinuses of mucous and debris that have previously accumulated. The endoscope is maintained in place to suction out all the material, and care should be taken to ensure this is not flushed down into the trachea around the endotracheal tube cuff. Finally, prior to removing the catheter, a local anesthetic (bupivicaine, 1 mg/kg for dogs; 0.2 mg/kg for cats) is injected at the level of the stenosis.

Complications of metallic stenting (MS) are further expanded upon. Success in maintaining patency with an uncovered metallic stent was recently reported in 67%

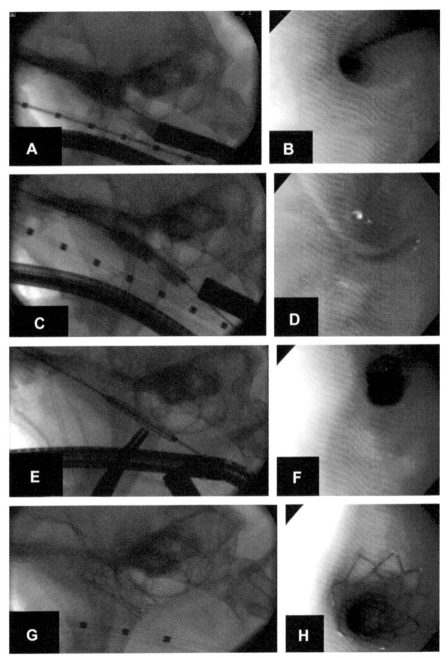

Fig. 5. Endoscopic and fluoroscopic images during the placement of an uncovered BEMS. (A) Fluoroscopic image during a contrast nasopharygraphy. Notice the marker catheter in the mouth being used for magnification. (B) Endoscopic image of the guide wire through the NPS. (C) Balloon passed over the wire during inflation of the NPS. Notice the waste of the stenosis as it breaks. (D) Endoscopic image of balloon dilation. (E) Placement of the BEMS over the guide wire prior to deployment. The hemostat is marking the location of the stenosis. (F) Endoscopic image of the stent prior to deployment ensuring it is across the caudal aspect of the NPS. (G) Fluroscopic image of the stent once it is deployed. (H) Endoscopic image of the stent after it is deployed showing coverage of the entire stenosis.

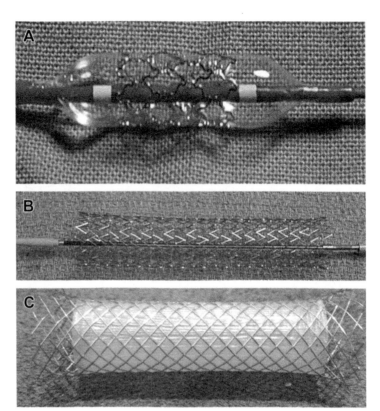

Fig. 6. Different types of stents used in the nasopharynx. (*A*) Balloon-expandable metallic stent during deployment. (*B*) Self-expanding metallic stent. (*C*) Partially-covered self-expanding metallic stent.

of dogs and cats, many of which had previously failed BD alone.[10] The remaining 33% of cases had tissue in-growth through the interstices of the uncovered MS, resulting in restenosis, and necessitating a covered metallic stent (CMS).[10]

Covered Metallic Stents

A CMS is placed exactly as described previously, depending on stent type (BEMS or SEMS). The only difference in the procedure is that they are often sutured to the soft palate to prevent stent migration since the stent does not incorporate into the naso-pharyngeal mucosa. The success of patency after a CMS is placed has been 100% in the cases it was placed,[10] and most of these patients had a CMS placed after tissue in-growth was found after BD and MS.

The median size of the stent used in cats was an 8 mm diameter and 20 mm length (range, 9–10 mm diameter × 16–34 mm length) and in dogs was 10 mm × 30 mm length (range, 7–16 mm diameter × 20–40 mm length).[10]

Temporary Tubing/Stenting

Using a piece of silicone tubing (like a chest tube-24 or 30 Fr) or a large bore catheter across the NPS after it is broken with balloon dilation or manual trauma is another option to consider. This can be done using fluoroscopic or endoscopic guidance, or using surgical assistance. In a recent study,[15] 15 cats with NPS had this procedure performed using silicone tubing and 14 of the 15 cats had resolution of the stenosis after the tubing was in place for 4 to 6 weeks. The author has tried this in only a small number of feline cases, and the tubing was poorly tolerated. It resulted in excessive gagging and swallowing, and persistent nasal discharge. When the tubing was removed, there was excessive inflammatory tissue around the ends of the tubing, and the owners were not happy with the quality of life while the tubing was in place. Long-term follow-up for success of NPS patency has not yet been observed at the time of writing this article. The NPS lesions typically seen in dogs are far more aggressive than that seen in cats, which is why they have such a high recurrence rate after BD and MS placement, often requiring a CMS. This would make one suspect that temporary stenting of dogs would not be as successful as that reported in cats.

A new stent that is being developed for NPS in canine and feline patients is a silicone-covered metallic stent that is retrievable. It is easy to deploy, like a typical SEMS, but has a retrieval mechanism so that endoscopically it can be removed after a period of time. This stent will be as well tolerated as typical SEMS, but easy to remove if needed. Other novel devices are being investigated for this condition also.

DISEASE COMPLICATIONS

Various complications are associated with each option and those are highlighted in **Table 1**. Most of these data are from the largest retrospective study to date, evaluating all minimally invasive treatment options for NPS in dogs and cats.[10] Tissue in-growth is the most common complication, seen in nearly 70% of patients after 1 BD procedure, and in 60% of patients that had between 1 and 3 BD procedures (100% of dogs and 50% of cats).[10] This percentage went down to 33% after MS placement.[10] For those with an imperforate membrane, tissue in-growth occurred in 67% of patients after MS, and only 25% of patients if the membrane was patent.[10] This would support that dogs and cats with imperforate membranes likely benefit from a CMS, as 0% of dogs or cats with a CMS had any tissue in-growth, and all were able to maintain patency of their nasopharynx.[10]

Complications associated with stents include

Tissue in-growth in 29% of patients (33% with MS; 0% CMS)
Chronic infections in 38% of patients (23% with MS; 54% CMS)
Stent fracture in 15% of patients (17% with MS; 0% with CMS)
Oral–nasal fistula development in 20% of patients (13% with MS; 27% with CMS)
Migration of the stent in 9% of patients (6.7% MS, 9% CMS)
Bending of the stent in 6% of patients (6.7% of MS; 0% CMS)
An exaggerated swallow in 6% of patients (6.7% MS, 0% CMS)
Necessary removal of the stent in 6% of patients (3.3% MS, 9% CMS)[10]

Oronasal fistula development can be handled in various different ways. Primary surgical closure is the most common approach. If this does not hold, then either a palatal flap can be performed or a covered stent can be placed across the hole to separate the 2 cavities. Both have been successful, but this complication can be costly and frustrating.

When location of the NPS was evaluated,[10] it was found that 67% of NPS cases in the proximal location, 100% of cases in the middle location, and 59% of cases in the caudal location had at least 1 complication ($P = .027$). Location of the NPS was not statistically associated with exaggerated swallow, fracture, bending, or need for removal, but was statistically associated with ONF (40% of middle location cases), in-growth (80% of middle cases), chronic infections (100% of middle cases), and migration (40% of middle cases).

Overall, in this study[10] 65% of all cases had at least 1 complication (70% BD, 70% MS, 55% CMS). There was no statistical correlation with sex, age, or the type of procedure performed. Tissue in-growth was the most common complication, and this was most common in the BD cases (59%–70%), and least common in the CMS cases (0%).

Seventy-six percent of cases were considered an ultimate success based on owners' interpretation of improved nasal airflow, decreased discharge, improved quality of life, and owner satisfaction.[10] Species was associated with outcome, as 87% of cats and 60% of dogs were considered ultimately successful ($P = .038$). Location was associated with outcome, as 90% of cases with a caudal NPS were successful, 67% of proximal cases, and 60% of middle cases. In this study, the median follow-up time was 24 months (range 6–109 months).[10]

PROGNOSIS/CONTROVERSIES

The condition of NPS is typically met with a good prognosis. The chance of some type of complication, usually minor, should be considered and discussed with the owners. With BD alone, a clinical success is reported to be 41% in the largest study to date,[10] and was up to 74% with a stent.[10] No dog in this study was successful with BD alone. Imperforate membranes are more likely to have complications and recurrent tissue in-growth after BD or MS, and in these cases, a CMS could be considered. The biggest complications to consider are tissue in-growth (59% BD, 33% MS, 0% CMS), chronic infections (23% MS, 54% CMS), and the development of an ONF (13% MS, 27% CMS). The cause of the ONF is not clear, but it is suspected that motion of the stent, which is most common for middle NPS lesions, could results in this lesion.

Using a temporary stent, as reported recently in a small series of cats,[15] has been met with great success in 1 report. The severity of the stenosis was not reported to be as dramatic as those that the author has seen. The author has tried this approach in 2 cats, and neither was successful. Recurrence occurred when the tubing was removed, and the tubing was poorly tolerated for the 6 weeks it was indwelling. This may be a different population of patients, as that report was from Europe. The author and colleagues are also looking at silicone-covered metallic stents that are easy to deploy, like an SEMS, and can be easily removed if necessary endoscopically.

SUMMARY

In summary, treatment of NPS using various minimally invasive options can be frustrating and can be met with a large number of complications, but most are usually successful if a stent is ultimately placed. These techniques are minimally invasive and relatively fast and simple. Complications should be discussed with all clients prior to considering, as cost: benefit needs to be considered. The largest series of 46 dogs and cats is made up of some of the worst and most severely affected cases that previously failed BD and were referred in a tertiary setting for a nasopharyngeal stent once the owners were limited financially. This means that this series is likely biased.[10] The biggest question for owners should be if they are willing to deal with some complications (62%) in order to get ultimately a good clinical outcome (74%). The alternative is living with the NPS.

REFERENCES

1. Billen F, Day MJ, Clercx C. Diagnosis of pharyngeal disorders in dogs: a retrospective study of 67 cases. J Small Anim Pract 2006;47:122–9.

2. Allen HS, Broussard J, Noone KE. Nasopharyngeal disease in cats; a retrospective study of 53 cases (1991-1998). J Am Anim Hosp Assoc 1999;35:457–61.
3. Novo RE, Kramek B. Surgical repair of nasopharyngeal stenosis in a cat using a stent. J Am Anim Hosp Assoc 1999;35:251–6.
4. Coolman BR, Marretta SM, McKiernan BC, et al. Choanal atresia and secondary nasopharyngeal stenosis in a dog. J Am Anim Hosp Assoc 1998;34:497–501.
5. Mitten RW. Nasopharyngeal stenosis in four cats. J Small Anim Pract 1988;29: 341–5.
6. Berent A, Weisse C, Todd K, et al. Use of a balloon-expandable metallic stent for treatment of nasopharyngeal stenosis in dogs and cats: six cases (2005-2007). J Am Vet Med Assoc 2008;233:1432–40.
7. Berent A, Kinns J, Weisse C. Balloon dilatation of nasopharyngeal stenosis in a dog. J Am Vet Med Assoc 2006;229:385–8.
8. Hunt GB, Perkins MC, Foster SF, et al. Nasopharyngeal disorder of dogs and cats: a review and retrospective study. Compend Contin Educ Pract Vet 2002; 24:184–98.
9. Cook A, Mankin K, Saunders A, et al. Palatal erosion and oronasal fistulation following covered nasophyangeal stent placement in two dogs. Ir Vet J 2013;66:8.
10. Burdick S, Berent A, Weisse C, et al. Evaluation of short and long term outcomes using various interventional treatment options for nasopharyngeal stenosis in 46 dogs and cats [Abstract]. Nashville (TN): Wiley-Blackwell; 2015.
11. Glaus TM, Tomsa K, Reusch CE. Balloon dilation for the treatment of chronic recurrent nasopharyngeal stenosis in a cat. J Small Anim Pract 2002;43:88–90.
12. Glaus TM, Gerber M, Tomsa K, et al. Reproducible and long-lasting success of balloon dilation of nasopharyngeal stenosis in cats. Vet Rec 2005;157:257–9.
13. Boswood A, Lamb CR, Brockman DJ, et al. Balloon dilatation of nasopharyngeal stenosis in a cat. Vet Radiol Ultrasound 2003;44:53–5.
14. Henderson SM, Day BM, Caney SM, et al. Investigation of nasal disease in the cat - a retrospective study of 77 cases. J Feline Med Surg 2004;6:245–57.
15. De Lorenzi D, Bertoncello D, Comastri S, et al. Treatment of acquired nasopharyngeal stenosis using a removalbe silicone stent. J Feline Med Surg 2015; 17(2):117–24.

Brachycephalic Syndrome

Gilles Dupré, Univ Prof Dr Med Vet*,
Dorothee Heidenreich, Dr Med Vet

KEYWORDS

- Brachycephalic airway obstructive syndrome • Soft palate • Laryngeal collapse
- Surgery

KEY POINTS

- Skull conformation anomalies in brachycephalic breeds lead to compression of nasal passages.
- Additional mucosal hyperplasia and secondary collapse of the upper airway contribute to a multilevel obstruction and the genesis of the so-called brachycephalic syndrome.
- Surgical treatments usually include widening of stenotic nares as well as various palatoplasty techniques to improve airflow through the rima glottidis.
- The overall prognosis for a significant improvement is excellent.

 Video content accompanies this article at http://www.vetsmall.theclinics.com

Brachycephalic syndrome (BS) is an established cause of respiratory distress in brachycephalic breeds.[1–3] Breeds most commonly affected are English and French bulldogs, pugs, and Boston terriers; however, Pekingese, Shih tzu, Cavalier King Charles Spaniels, Boxers, Dogue de Bordeaux, and Bullmastiffs are also categorized as brachycephalic dogs.[4] Most owners report heat, stress and exercise intolerance, snoring, inspiratory dyspnea, and in severe cases, cyanosis and even syncopal episodes. Sleep apneas can be observed,[5] and occasionally gastrointestinal signs such as vomiting and regurgitation.

ANATOMIC AND PATHOPHYSIOLOGIC CHANGES OBSERVED IN BRACHYCEPHALIC BREEDS
Skull Conformation Anomalies

Brachycephalic breeds have a shorter and wider skull compared with mesaticephalic and dolichicephalic breeds,[6,7] which leads to a compressed nasal passage[8] and

Disclosure Statement: The authors have nothing to disclose.
Department for Small Animal and Equine, Vetmeduni Vienna, Veterinary Medicine University, Veterinärplatz 1, A-1210 Vienna, Austria
* Corresponding author.
E-mail address: Gilles.dupre@vetmeduni.ac.at

altered pharyngeal anatomy.[9–11] In addition, pugs are reported to have a dorsal rotation of the maxillary bone, miniscule or absent frontal sinuses,[12,13] a ventral orientation of the olfactorial bulb,[14] and altogether, a shorter craniofacial skull measurement than French and English bulldogs.[12,14–17]

This dorsal rotation has been discussed as a potential cause for aberrant nasopharyngeal turbinates, which are also more commonly reported in pugs (**Figs. 1** and **2**).[3,12,18–20]

Soft Tissues Changes

Stenotic nares

One typical and easily recognized primary anatomic component of brachycephalic syndrome.

BS-affected dogs have stenotic nares, which reduce each nostril to a vertical slit (**Fig. 3**).

Soft palate hyperplasia

Although the literature used to emphasize an elongated soft palate,[2,18,21] fluttering, and obstructing the rima glottidis as a primary component of BS, recent radiographic, computed tomography (CT), and histologic examinations demonstrated an additional pathologic thickening of the soft palate, which might play a major role in the nasopharyngeal obstruction.[3,13,22–27] One study[22] demonstrated a positive correlation between the thickness of the soft palate and the severity of the clinical signs. A recent study using CT evaluation of airway dimension showed a significantly thicker soft palate in French bulldogs compared with pugs but no free airway space dorsal to the soft palate in 81% of pugs.[13] In addition to soft palate hyperplasia, CT and endoscopic studies reported hyperplasia of the nasopharyngeal mucosa,[28,29] hypertrophy and eversion of the tonsils,[30] and an overlong and thickened tongue (macroglossia), which further displaces the soft palate dorsally.[31]

Laryngeal, Tracheal, and Bronchial Anomalies

Laryngeal diseases

Laryngeal diseases associated with BS are thought to be mainly secondary to the turbulent airflow and chronic high negative pressures in the pharynx.[2,21,23,32,33] They include

- Mucosal edema
- Everted laryngeal saccules (ELS)
- Laryngeal collapse

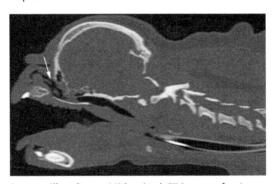

Fig. 1. Dorsal rotation maxillary bone. Midsagittal CT image of a 4-year-old pug depicting dorsal rotation (*arrow*) of the maxillary bone.

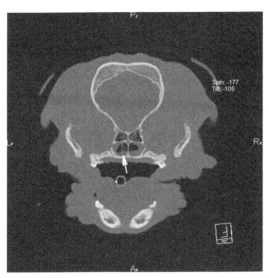

Fig. 2. Aberrant turbinates. Transverse CT image of a French bulldog depicting aberrant nasopharyngeal turbinates (*arrow*).

In one early classification, ELS were considered the first stage of laryngeal collapse[34] (**Fig. 4**). Stage 2 was characterized by a medial displacement of the cuneiform processes of the arytenoid cartilages, and stage 3 by a collapse of the corniculate processes with loss of the dorsal arch of the rima glottidis. Altogether, the incidence of laryngeal collapse varies from 50%[35,36] to as many as 95%[37] in BS-affected dogs. Studies report that the size of the rima glottidis is smaller in pugs[38] and that they are also significantly more often affected by severe laryngeal collapse than French bulldogs.[39] In this breed, the arytenoid cartilages can even invert into the laryngeal lumen as a consequence of lack of rigidity (chondromalacia), which makes the larynx incapable to withstand high negative pharyngeal pressures[23] (Video 1).

Tracheal and bronchial anomalies
Tracheal hypoplasia,[2,18,40] as defined as a tracheal diameter (TD) to the thoracic inlet (TI) ratio (TD:TI) less than 0.2 in nonbrachycephliac and less than 0.16 in

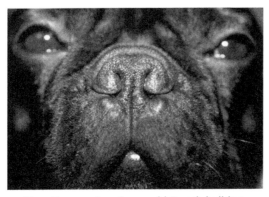

Fig. 3. Stenotic nares. Stenotic nares in a 2-year-old French bulldog.

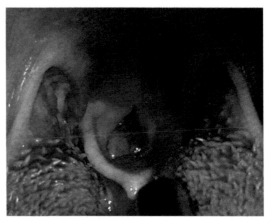

Fig. 4. Everted laryngeal saccules. Laryngoscopic view of the rima glottides of a dog a French bulldog with stage 1 laryngeal collapse with everted laryngeal saccules.

brachycephalic dogs,[41] has been described in 13% of BS-affected dogs.[10,42] The English bulldog has the highest incidence of tracheal hypoplasia among brachycephalic breeds, and tracheal hypoplasia in this breed has been defined as a TD:TI ratio of less than 0.12. Although tracheal hypoplasia increases airway resistance, its contribution to the syndrome is likely minimal.[3]

Bronchial collapse was found to be significantly correlated to the severity of the laryngeal collapse ($P = .45$), and pugs were found to be most severely affected. Left-side bronchi were generally more affected by bronchial collapse (52.1%) than the right, with the cranial left bronchus most commonly collapsed.[37] Whether the etiology is loss of rigidity (chondromalacia), increased negative pressure or compression within the chest remains to be investigated (Video 2).

Gastroesophageal Diseases Associated with Brachycephalic Syndrome

Dysphagia, vomiting, and regurgitation are common clinical signs in brachycephalic breeds,[32] and investigation of dogs affected by BS showed concurrent esophageal, gastric, or duodenal anomalies.[43] The negative intrathoracic pressures generated by increased inspiratory effort[44–47] is believed to be a major cause of gastroesophageal reflux. The associated regurgitation and vomiting can contribute to upper esophageal, pharyngeal, and laryngeal inflammation.[48] French bulldogs exhibit significantly more often and more severe digestive signs than pugs.[39,49]

DIAGNOSIS

Diagnosis is usually based on owners' reports, clinical examination, and diagnostic imaging.

Clinical Diagnosis

Snoring, inspiratory dyspnea, cyanosis, and in the most severe cases, syncopal episodes are most often reported by owners. On inspection, stenotic nares and inspiratory efforts with even abdominal breathing can be observed. A particular attention shall be paid to respiratory sounds.

Whereas snoring is most likely caused by air turbulences in the oro-pharyngeal region, the high-pitch sound associated with extreme inspiratory effort is related to more severe airway compromise when turbulent air is passing through the collapsed larynx or nasopharynx.

Diagnostic Imaging

Radiographic, fluoroscopic, CT, and endoscopic studies all contribute to the evaluation of the static and dynamic obstruction of the respiratory tract.[8,12,13,22,23,50] In a clinical practice setting, a proper evaluation of BS patients should include at least neck and thoracic radiographs, and endoscopic examination of the upper airways.

- Thoracic radiographs are performed to document secondary heart or lung diseases and to rule out aspiration pneumonia. Also, on occasion a sliding hiatal hernia can incidentally be found on a lateral radiograph.
- Lateral radiographs of the neck (when CT is not available) can help to assess the soft palate thickness as defined by the soft tissue density present between the nasopharynx and oropharynx.[1]
- CT evaluation of the head and neck allows a detailed assessment of the nostrils, vestibule, nasal cavity, and nasopharynx and oropharynx (**Fig. 5**).[12,13,22]
- Endoscopic examination provides more information on the dynamic changes within the upper airways:
  - With the dog intubated, retrograde rhinoscopy performed with a 120° rigid scope or a flexible endoscope allows for good evaluation of nasopharyngeal tissue hyperplasia and collapse as well as for the presence of aberrant turbinates (**Fig. 6**, Videos 3 and 4).
  - With the dog extubated, a laryngoscopic examination can expose ELS and also help evaluate laryngeal dynamics. With laryngeal collapse, lack of abduction during inspiration or even paradoxic movements of the arytenoid cartilages can occur. In pugs and other dogs affected by laryngeal chondromalacia, the dorsal border of the cuneiform process of the arytenoid cartilages can even invert into the laryngeal lumen (Video 5).

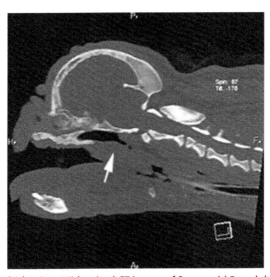

Fig. 5. Soft palate thickening. Midsagittal CT image of 2-year-old French bulldog with thickening of the soft palate (*arrow*).

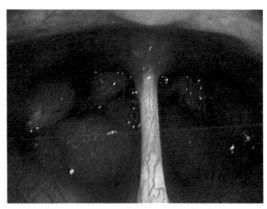

Fig. 6. Nasopharyngeal turbinates. Images of a retrograde rhinoscopy displaying aberrant nasopharyngeal turbinates.

CONTROVERSY REGARDING THE GENESIS OF BRACHYCEPHALIC SYNDROME

The genesis of BS is thought to be due to anatomic changes which lead to increased inspiratory resistance.[32,42,51,52] With significant negative pressure, the soft tissues are drawn into the lumen resulting in collapse of the upper airway.[23,32] Eversion of the laryngeal saccules, nasopharyngeal collapse, and laryngeal collapse, are suspected to contribute to clinical signs and further deterioration of BS, which might ultimately cause syncopal episodes and death from suffocation.[42,52]

Although, in the past, an overlong soft palate fluttering in the rima glottidis has been considered as the main cause of BS, it remains difficult to estimate the greatest contributor to the clinical signs. The nose is known to be the greatest source of flow resistance in the total airway system,[53,54] and rhinomanometric studies confirm that intranasal resistance is significantly higher in brachycephalic dogs compared with normal dogs.[55,56] The major upper airway obstruction was postulated to be intranasal secondary to aberrant turbinates[12] or located in the compressed nasopharynx.[22] But late CT studies comparing pugs and French bulldogs found that the smallest airway space is located dorsal to the soft palate even in dogs with aberrant nasopharyngeal turbinates.[13] Additionally, aberrant turbinates were also described in clinically normal English bulldogs,[57] which means that the contribution of the aberrant turbinates to BS needs to be more thoroughly evaluated.

Although laryngeal collapse has usually been considered to be associated with progression of the disease, a significant correlation between age and severity of laryngeal collapse was demonstrated only recently.[39] In another study including pugs and English and French bulldogs with stage 1 laryngeal collapse, no correlation between Glottic index and age or weight could be demonstrated.[38] Finally, the overall postoperative prognosis of BS was not affected by the grade of laryngeal collapse in 2 recent studies.[21,39]

Overall, although it is clear that air cannot flow through the nose as long as the nostrils are obstructed, it remains uncertain which part of the obstructed airway—nasal cavity, nasopharynx or rima glottis—is most responsible for the clinical signs associated with BS. In that regard, the effect of soft palate resection might be due to the opening of the nasopharyngeal space and not to the relief of the rima glottidis obstruction.

TREATMENT OF BRACHYCEPHALIC SYNDROME
Medical Therapy

Patients presented with acute signs of respiratory distress should be treated accordingly with cooling, tranquilizers, oxygen therapy, and anti-inflammatory drugs. Whenever digestive signs are observed in dogs with BS, medical treatment including inhibition of hydrogen ion secretion and gastric prokinetic drugs is recommended before and immediately after surgery.

Surgical Therapy

Timing

According to the pathophysiology of the syndrome, relief of the proximally located obstruction should be attempted early to prevent deterioration or possibly reverse tissue collapse,[10,42,58] but the optimal time to correct upper airway obstruction has not been determined and was recommended to be performed after the age of 6 months. Recent studies suggest that improvement in clinical signs is still obtained when surgery is performed on mature and middle-aged dogs.[39]

Stenotic Nares

Several surgical options have been described for correction of stenotic nares: amputation of the ala nasi,[59,60] various alaplasty techniques, alapexy,[61] and vestibuloplasty.

Alaplasty is the most used procedure and consists of the excision of a wedge of the ala nasi with primary closure of the defect. This wedge excision can be made vertically, horizontally,[58,62] or laterally.[10,42,63] Incisions are made with a No. 11 or 15 scalpel blade or alternatively with a punch.[64] Two to 4 simple interrupted sutures, using absorbable monofilament material, are placed to appose the wedge margins. Hemorrhage resolves quickly when the wound is sutured (Video 6).

Vestibuloplasty has been advocated instead of alaplasty to further improve airflow.[65] It involves the dorsomedial and caudal portion of the ala and results in a wide and open vestibule.

Turbinectomy

Turbinectomy[66] and its laser-assisted variation (LATE)[67] are aimed at removal of malformed obstructive parts of the ventral and medial nasal turbinates. The LATE, combined with vestibuloplasty and staphylectomy, resulted in a decrease of 55% of intranasal resistance 3 to 6 months after surgery compared with preoperative values.[55] Studies show partial regrowth of the removed turbinates but with less mucosal contact points.[68] The long-term positive effects of turbinectomy on intranasal resistance and adverse effects on thermoregulation require further investigation.

Elongated–Hyperplastic Soft Palate

Common surgical techniques for correction of elongated soft palate are aimed at shortening the soft palate by simple resection of its caudal portion (staphylectomy), to prevent it from obstructing the rima glottidis on inspiration. Different landmarks have been recommended, varying from the tip of epiglottis,[32,62,69–71] or the middle to caudal aspect of the palatine tonsils.[10,33,69,71,72]

During staphylectomy, the caudal border of the soft palate is grasped and held with Allis forceps or stay sutures,[70,73] and resection of excessive length of soft palate can be performed with a scalpel blade,[5,58,70] scissors,[32,42,62,74] monopolar electrocoagulation,[58,69,75] carbon dioxide laser,[2,71,75–77] diode laser,[75] or bipolar sealing device (Ligasure, Valleylab, Covidien, Boulder, Colorado).[73,77]

As these palate-trimming techniques may not address the soft palate hyperplasia, techniques designed to more extensively shorten and thin the soft palate have been described.[24,73,75,78,79] The folded flap palatoplasty (FFP) has been developed to correct both the excessive length and excessive thickness of the soft palate, therefore relieving also nasopharyngeal obstruction.[24,78,79] In this technique, the soft palate is made thinner by excision of a portion of its oropharyngeal mucosa and underlying soft tissues. In addition, the palate is made shorter by being folded onto itself until the caudal nasopharyngeal opening is readily visible transorally (**Box 1**, **Figs. 7–9**, Video 7).

Postoperative adverse effects or pharyngo-nasal regurgitation have not been observed with the folded flap palatoplasty.[73,75,79] Whatever technique is chosen, a telescope and high-definition camera system for magnification and illumination of the surgical field (VITOM TM, Karl Storz Endoscopy, Tuttlingen, Germany) are helpful (**Fig. 10**).

Surgical Treatments for Laryngeal Diseases

Everted laryngeal saccules

Excision of ELS has been described using electrocautery, scissors, tonsil snares or laryngeal biopsy cup forceps.[1,10,21,32,42,62,69,72] In 1 study reevaluating ELS after single side resection, no regression of the nonremoved site despite treatment of nares and soft palate was found.[80] Altogether, whether resection of the ELS is needed remains questionable. In several recent BS outcome studies, in which nares and palates were corrected but ELS were either not or rarely addressed, outcomes appeared to be similar to studies in which ELS were excised.[29,75,79] Also, complications such as laryngeal webbing and regrowth can occur.[81,82] With this in mind, the authors only recommend removal of ELS when the eversion contributes significantly to the obstruction.

Laryngeal collapse

As laryngeal collapse is suspected to be secondary to proximal airway obstruction, first address the proximal obstruction areas (ie, nares and soft palate), as this may obviate the need to treat the collapse.[2,3,21,23,33,83] In the author's experience, surgical

---

Box 1
The folded flap palatoplasty: surgical technique

- The head is restrained and the mouth kept open. The tongue is pulled rostrally and maintained with a malleable retractor connected to an articulated arm.

- The caudal edge of the soft palate is grasped with forceps and retracted rostrally and dorsally into the oropharynx, until the caudal opening of the nasopharynx can be visualized.

- The contact point on the ventral mucosa of the soft palate is marked, as this represents the proximal cut of the soft palate.

- The ventral mucosa of the soft palate is then incised in a trapezoidal shape from this mark rostrally to the free edge of the soft palate caudally.

- Laterally, the sides of the trapeze passed just medially to the tonsils.

- The soft tissues under the cut portion of the soft palate are excised together with part of the levator veli palatini muscle.

- The caudal edge of the soft palate is retracted rostrally and is sutured folded on itself with simple interrupted monofilament absorbable sutures.

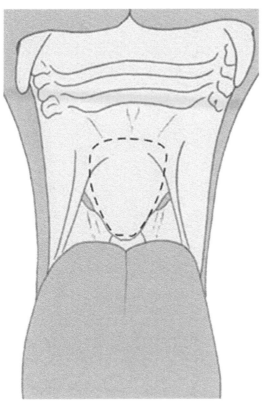

Fig. 7. Folded flap palatoplasty: incision lines in the oral mucosa for the thinning process of soft palate hyperplasia.

treatment of laryngeal collapse is considered only when clinical signs do not improve after appropriate treatment of the nares and soft palate. Partial laryngectomy as described earlier[69] has been found to be associated with unacceptably high (50%) mortality rates, and is no longer recommended.[72] Laser-assisted partial arytenoidectomy as recommended for treatment of laryngeal paralysis might provide some relief[84] but needs to be further investigated. Alternatively, arytenoid lateralization is a valid option for dogs with sufficient mineralization of the laryngeal cartilages.[33,44,85] On the contrary, its efficacy is questionable in pugs and dogs suffering from chrondromalacia when arytenoid cartilages have a tendency to inwardly rotate during inspiration (pugs).[21,23] If there is inefficient relief of airway obstruction after the previously mentioned procedures, a permanent tracheostomy can be attempted as a palliative option.[1,10,32,42,58,86]

Removal of other hyperplastic tissues

Excision of the palatine tonsils has been recommended when they seem to contribute to pharyngeal obstruction.[42,69,74] However, the advantage of tonsillectomy warrants further investigation.[30,32,62] Similarly, excision of redundant soft tissues located in the pharynx, especially in its dorsal aspect, has been suggested,[62] but more data are needed to evaluate which of the pharyngeal tissues are involved in the obstruction process and the optimal surgical method to remove the hyperplastic tissue.

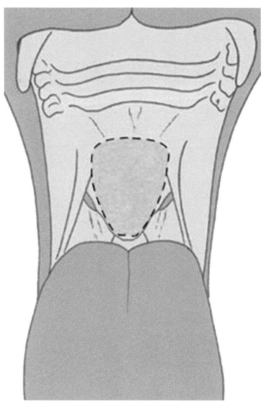

Fig. 8. Folded flap palatoplasty: end of dissection of the soft palate. The yellow area depicts the removed oral part of the soft palate.

Tracheostomy

Although it has been advocated in the past, a preoperative temporary tracheostomy[1,69,87] is not necessary. Postoperative temporary tracheostomy has been reported in the past in 5% to 28% of cases.[21,29,58,79,88] As the complication rate of temporary tracheostomy in brachycephalic dogs is very high (86% in 1 study)[89] it should therefore be reserved for cases not responding to routine postoperative care.

Postoperative Care

The challenge during the postoperative period is to enable adequate airflow in a not yet fully awake patient with potentially swollen airway mucosa. It is critical that BS dogs are monitored constantly after extubation to determine if ventilation is inadequate.

Several methods can be combined or used independently to help relieve upper airway obstruction or improve ventilation after surgical repair:

- The dog can be recovered with the upper jaw hung up, which allows the lower jaw to drop, further opening the airway (**Fig. 11**).
- Increasing the oxygen delivery—placement of a small nasotracheal tube immediately after surgery but before the dog is awake is a very simple technique of insufflating oxygen, allowing oxygen delivery beyond the rima glottis.[3,90]

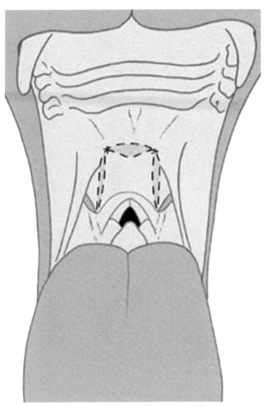

Fig. 9. Folded flap palatoplasty: schematic view showing folding of thinned soft palate upon itself.

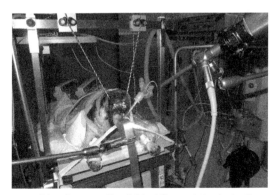

Fig. 10. Surgery set-up with telescope. For folded flap palatoplasty, the mouth of the dog is kept open, and the tongue is pushed down using a malleable retractor. Magnification is provided with the Exoscope (VITOM TM, Karl Storz Endoscopy, Tuttlingen, Germany).

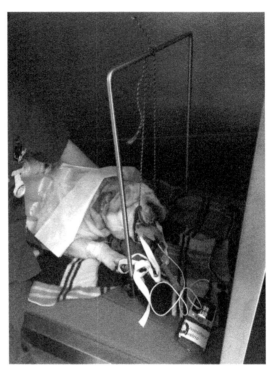

Fig. 11. Patient recovery after BS surgery. Bulldog recovering from anesthesia with the upper jaw hung to help open the mouth to improve oxygenation.

PROGNOSIS

It is difficult to gain an accurate perspective of the prognosis for individual dogs afflicted with BS.[2,21,33,58,64,71,76,91] Most studies evaluating outcome after BS surgery are retrospective in nature, and compare results in different breeds with various combinations of treatments and reconstructive techniques. In addition, these studies compare outcomes with surgical treatments performed at variable patient ages and by different surgeons, using different grading systems,[24,60,73,75] Furthermore, it is difficult to compare the postoperative outcome in these various studies, because there is often a mismatch between the owners' perception of their pets clinical disability and the severity of the clinical signs.[92] A recent study compared preoperative and postoperative treatments in different breeds that underwent the same diagnostic work-up, treatment, and evaluation methods.[39] Despite inherent study limitations, late studies report that around 90% of BS dogs are significantly improved with surgery.[2,24,29,39,75] This is better than earlier reports. Similarly, perioperative mortality rates have improved from around 15% in earlier reports[58,91] to less than 4% in more recent studies.[2,24,29,73,75] Postoperative improvement is most often observed immediately after surgery.[24,29] Some studies report long-term recurrence of clinical signs in up to 100% of cases, although 89% of dogs still remain improved compared with their preoperative status.[21] In other studies, clinical grades improved in the first 2 weeks after folded flap palatoplasty[24,39] and remained the same over the following period (mean 12–22 months).

SUMMARY

Animals presenting with BS suffer of multilevel obstruction of the airways and second-ary soft tissue collapse. Despite progresses achieved through advanced diagnostic modalities such as CT and endoscopy, the main contributor to the increased inspira-tory efforts remains to be found. Recent studies suggest that postoperative prognosis is good even in middle-aged dogs.

SUPPLEMENTARY DATA

Supplementary data related to this article can be found at http://dx.doi.org/10.1016/j. cvsm.2016.02.002.

REFERENCES

1. Hendricks JC. Brachycephalic airway syndrome. Vet Clin North Am Small Anim Pract 1992;22:1145–53.
2. Riecks TW, Birchard SJ, Stephens JA. Surgical correction of brachycephalic syn-drome in dogs: 62 cases (1991-2004). J Am Vet Med Assoc 2007;230:1324–8.
3. Dupré G, Findji L, Oechtering G. Brachycephalic airway syndrome. In: Monnet E, editor. Small animal soft tissue surgery. Ames (IA): Wiley-Blackwell; 2012. p. 167–83.
4. Meola SD. Brachycephalic airway syndrome. Top Companion Anim Med 2013;28: 91–6.
5. Farquharson J, Smith DW. Resection of the soft palate in the dog. J Am Vet Med Assoc 1942;100:427–30.
6. Stockard CR. The genetic and endocrinic basis for differences in form and behavior. Am Anat Memoir 1941;19:775.
7. Evans HE. The skeleton. In: Evans HE, editor. Millers' anatomy of the dog. Phila-delphia: Saunders; 1993. p. 122–218.
8. Schuenemann R, Oechtering GU. Inside the brachycephalic nose: intranasal mucosal contact points. J Am Anim Hosp Assoc 2014;50:149–58.
9. Arrighi S, Pichetto M, Roccabianca P, et al. The anatomy of the dog soft palate. I. Histological evaluation of the caudal soft palate in mesaticephalic breeds. Anat Rec (Hoboken) 2011;294:1261–6.
10. Wykes PM. Brachycephalic airway obstructive syndrome. Probl Vet Med 1991;3: 188–97.
11. Trappler M, Moore K. Canine brachycephalic airway syndrome: pathophysiology, diagnosis, and nonsurgical management. Compend Contin Educ Vet 2011;33(5): E1–4.
12. Oechtering TH, Oechtering GU, Nöller C. Strukturelle besonderheiten der nase brachyzephaler hunderassen in der computertomographie. Tierärztl Prax 2007; 35:177–87.
13. Heidenreich D, Gradner G, Kneissl S, et al. Nasopharyngeal dimensions from computed tomography of pugs and french bulldogs with brachycephalic airway syndrome. Vet Surg 2016;45(1):83–90.
14. Hussein AK, Sullivan M, Penderis J. Effect of brachycephalic, mesaticephalic, and dolichocephalic head conformations on olfactory bulb angle and orientation in dogs as determined by use of in vivo magnetic resonance imaging. Am J Vet Res 2012;73:946–51.
15. Hennet PR, Harvey CE. Craniofacial development and growth in the dog. J Vet Dent 1992;9:11–8.

16. Hussein AK. MRI mensuration of the canine head: the effect of head conformation on the shape and dimensions of the facial and cranial regions and their components [PhD Thesis]. Glasgow (United Kingdom): University of Glasgow; 2012.

17. Regodon S, Vivo JM, Franco A, et al. Craniofacial angle in dolicho-, meso- and brachycephalic dogs: radiological determination and application. Anat Anz 1993;175(4):361–3.

18. Ginn JA, Kumar MS, McKiernan BC, et al. Nasopharyngeal turbinates in brachycephalic dogs and cats. J Am Anim Hosp Assoc 2008;44:243–9.

19. Billen F, Day M, Clercx C. Diagnosis of pharyngeal disorders in dogs: a retrospective study of 67 cases. J Small Anim Pract 2006;47:122–9.

20. Heidenreich DC, Dupré G. The nasopharyngeal space in brachycephalic dogs: a computed tomographic comparison of Pugs and French Bulldogs. In: Proceedings 24th ECVS Annual Meeting. Berlin (Germany): Vet Surg; 2015. p. E20, 44(5).

21. Torrez CV, Hunt GB. Results of surgical correction of abnormalities associated with brachycephalic airway obstruction syndrome in dogs in Australia. J Small Anim Pract 2006;47:150–4.

22. Grand JG, Bureau S. Structural characteristics of the soft palate and meatus nasopharyngeus in brachycephalic and non-brachycephalic dogs analysed by CT. J Small Anim Pract 2011;52:232–9.

23. Dupré G, Poncet C. Respiratory system - brachycephalic upper airways syndrome. In: Bojrab MJ, editor. Mechanisms of diseases in small animal surgery. 3rd edition. Jackson (WY): Teton New Media; 2010. p. 298–301.

24. Findji L, Dupré G. Folded flap palatoplasty for treatment of elongated soft palates in 55 dogs. Eur J Companion Anim Pract 2009;19:125–32.

25. Pichetto M, Arrighi S, Roccabianca P, et al. The anatomy of the dog soft palate. II. Histological evaluation of the caudal soft palate in brachycephalic breeds with grade I brachycephalic airway obstructive syndrome. Anat Rec (Hoboken) 2011;294:1267–72.

26. Pichetto M, Arrighi S, Gobbetti M, et al. The anatomy of the dog soft palate. III. Histological evaluation of the caudal soft palate in brachycephalic neonates. Anat Rec (Hoboken) 2015;298:618–23.

27. Crosse KR, Bray JP, Orbell G, et al. Histological evaluation of the soft palate in dogs affected by brachycephalic obstructive airway syndrome. N Z Vet J 2015; 63(6):319–25.

28. Oechtering GU, Hueber JP, Kiefer I, et al. Laser assisted turbinectomy (LATE): a novel approach to brachycephalic airway syndrome. In: Proceedings 16th ECVS Meeting. Dublin (Ireland): Vet Surg; 2007. p. E11, 36(4).

29. Poncet CM, Dupré GP, Freiche VG, et al. Long-term results of upper respiratory syndrome surgery and gastrointestinal tract medical treatment in 51 brachycephalic dogs. J Small Anim Pract 2006;47(3):137–42.

30. Fasanella FJ, Shivley JM, Wardlaw JL, et al. Brachycephalic airway obstructive syndrome in dogs: 90 cases (1991-2008). J Am Vet Med Assoc 2010;237: 1048–51.

31. Fox MW. Developmental abnormalities of the canine skull. Can J Comp Med Vet Sci 1963;27(9):219–22.

32. Koch DA, Arnold S, Hubler M, et al. Brachycephalic syndrome in dogs. Comp Cont Ed 2003;25(1):48–55.

33. Pink JJ, Doyle RS, Hughes JML, et al. Laryngeal collapse in seven brachycephalic puppies. J Small Anim Pract 2006;47(3):131–5.

34. Leonard HC. Collapse of the larynx and adjacent structures in the dog. J Am Vet Med Assoc 1960;137:360–3.

35. Wilson FD, Rajendran EI, David G. Staphylotomy in a dachshund. Indian Vet J 1960;37:639–42.

36. Wegner W. Genetisch bedingte zahnanomalien. Prakt Tierarzt 1987;68(5):19–22.

37. De Lorenzi D, Bertoncello D, Drigo M. Bronchial abnormalities found in a consecutive series of 40 brachycephalic dogs. J Am Vet Med Assoc 2009;235(7): 835–40.

38. Caccamo R, Buracco P, La Rosa G, et al. Glottic and skull indices in canine brachycephalic airway obstructive syndrome. BMC Vet Res 2014;10:12.

39. Haimel G, Dupré G. Brachycephalic airway syndrome: a comparative study between pugs and French bulldogs. J Small Anim Pract 2015;56(12):714–9.

40. Coyne BE, Fingland RB. Hypoplasia of the trachea in dogs: 103 cases (1974-1990). J Am Vet Med Assoc 1992;201(5):768–72.

41. Harvey CE, Fink EA. Tracheal diameter: analysis of radiographic measurements in brachycephalic and nonbrachycephalic dogs. J Am Anim Hosp Assoc 1982; 18:570–6.

42. Aron DN, Crowe DT. Upper airway obstruction. general principles and selected conditions in the dog and cat. Vet Clin North Am Small Anim Pract 1985;15(5): 891–917.

43. Poncet CM, Dupré GP, Freiche VG, et al. Prevalence of gastrointestinal tract lesions in 73 brachycephalic dogs with upper respiratory syndrome. J Small Anim Pract 2005;46(6):273–9.

44. Ducarouge B. Le syndrome obstructif des voies respiratoies supèrieures chez les chiens brachycèphales. etude clinique à propos de 27 cas [Thesis]. Lyon (France): University Lyon; 2002.

45. Hardie EM, Ramirez O, Clary EM, et al. Abnormalities of the thoracic bellows: Stress fractures of the ribs and hiatal hernia. J Vet Intern Med 1998;12(4):279–87.

46. Hunt GB, O'Brien C, Kolenc G, et al. Hiatal hernia in a puppy. Aust Vet J 2002; 80(11):685–6.

47. Miles KG, Pope ER, Jergens AE. Paraesophageal hiatal hernia and pyloric obstruction in a dog. J Am Vet Med Assoc 1988;193(11):1437–9.

48. White DR, Heavner SB, Hardy SM, et al. Gastroesophageal reflux and eustachian tube dysfunction in an animal model. Laryngoscope 2002;112(6):955–61.

49. Roedler FS, Pohl S, Oechtering GU. How does severe brachycephaly affect dog's lives? Results of a structured preoperative owner questionnaire. Vet J 2013;198: 606–10.

50. Rubin JA, Holt DE, Reetz JA, et al. Signalment, clinical presentation, concurrent diseases, and diagnostic findings in 28 dogs with dynamic pharyngeal collapse (2008-2013). J Vet Intern Med 2015;29:815–21.

51. Leonard HC. Eversion of the lateral ventricles of the larynx in dogs - five cases. J Am Vet Med Assoc 1957;131:83–4.

52. Cook WR. Observations on the upper respiratory tract of the dog and cat. J Small Anim Pract 1964;5:309–29.

53. Ohnishi T, Ogura JH. Partitioning of pulmonary resistance in the dog. Laryngoscope 1969;79(11):1847–78.

54. Negus VE, Oram S, Banks DC. Effect of respiratory obstruction on the arterial and venous circulation in animals and man. Thorax 1970;25(1):1–10.

55. Hueber J. Impulse oscillometric examination of intranasal airway resistance before and after laser assisted turbinectomy for treatment of brachycephalic airway syndrome in the dog [Thesis]. Leipzig (Germany): University of Leipzig; 2008.

56. Lippert JP, Reinhold P, Smith HJ, et al. Geometry and function of the canine nose: how does the function change when the form is changed? Pneumologie 2010; 64(7):452–3.

57. Vilaplana Grosso F, Haar GT, Boroffka SA. Gender, weight, and age effects on prevalence of caudal aberrant nasal turbinates in clinically healthy english bulldogs: a computed tomographic study and classification. Vet Radiol Ultrasound 2015;56(5):486–93.

58. Harvey CE. Soft palate resection in brachycephalic dogs. II. J Am Anim Hosp Assoc 1982;18:538–44.

59. Trader RL. Nose operation. J Am Vet Med Assoc 1949;114:210–1.

60. Huck JL, Stanley BJ, Hauptman JG. Technique and outcome of nares amputation (trader's technique) in immature shih tzus. J Am Vet Med Assoc 2008;44(2):82–5.

61. Ellison GW. Alapexy: an alternative technique for repair of stenotic nares in dogs. J Am Vet Med Assoc 2004;40(6):484–9.

62. Hobson HP. Brachycephalic syndrome. Semin Vet Med Surg (Small Anim) 1995; 10(2):109–14.

63. Nelson A. Upper respiratory system. In: Slatter DG, editor. Textbook of small animal surgery. 2nd edition. Philadelphia: Saunders; 1993. p. 733–76.

64. Trostel CT, Frankel DJ. Punch resection alaplasty technique in dogs and cats with stenotic nares: 14 cases. J Am Vet Med Assoc 2010;46(1):5–11.

65. Oechtering GU, Schuenemann R. Brachycephalics-trapped in man-made misery? Proceedings AVSTS Meeting. Cambridge (United Kingdom): 2010. p. 28.

66. Tobias KM. Stenotic nares. In: Tobias KM, editor. Manual of soft tissue surgery. Oxford (United Kingdom): Wiley-Blackwell; 2010. p. 401–6.

67. Oechtering GU, Hueber JP, Oechtering TH, et al. Laser assisted turbinectomy (LATE): treating brachycephalic airway distress at its intranasal origin. In: Proceedings ACVS Meeting. Chicago (IL): Vet Surg; 2007. p. E18, 36(6).

68. Schuenemann R, Oechtering G. Inside the brachycephalic nose: conchal regrowth and mucosal contact points after laser-assisted turbinectomy. J Am Anim Hosp Assoc 2014;50:237–46.

69. Harvey CE, Venker-von Haagan A. Surgical management of pharyngeal and laryngeal airway obstruction in the dog. Vet Clin North Am Small Anim Pract 1975;5:515–35.

70. Bright RM, Wheaton LG. A modified surgical technique for elongated soft palate in dogs. J Am Vet Med Assoc 1983;19:288.

71. Davidson EB, Davis MS, Campbell GA, et al. Evaluation of carbon dioxide laser and conventional incisional techniques for resection of soft palates in brachycephalic dogs. J Am Vet Med Assoc 2001;219(6):776–81.

72. Harvey CE. Review of results of airway obstruction surgery in the dog. J Small Anim Pract 1983;24(9):555–9.

73. Brdecka DJ, Rawlings CA, Perry AC, et al. Use of an electrothermal, feedback-controlled, bipolar sealing device for resection of the elongated portion of the soft palate in dogs with obstructive upper airway disease. J Am Vet Med Assoc 2008;233(8):1265–9.

74. Singleton WB. Partial velum palatiectomy for relief of dyspnea in brachycephalic breeds. J Small Anim Pract 1962;3:215–6.

75. Dunié-Mérigot A, Bouvy B, Poncet C. Comparative use of CO_2 laser, diode laser and monopolar electrocautery for resection of the soft palate in dogs with brachycephalic airway obstruction syndrome. Vet Rec 2010;167:700–4.

76. Clark GN, Sinibaldi KR. Use of a carbon dioxide laser for treatment of elongated soft palate in dogs. J Am Vet Med Assoc 1994;204(11):1779–81.

77. Brdecka D, Rawlings C, Howerth E, et al. A histopathological comparison of two techniques for soft palate resection in normal dogs. J Am Vet Med Assoc 2007; 43(1):39–44.

78. Dupré G, Findji L. Nouvelle technique chirurgicale: La palatoplastie modifiée chez le chien. Nouveau Prat Vet 2004;20:553–6.

79. Findji L, Dupré GP. Folded flap palatoplasty for treatment of elongated soft palates in 55 dogs. Vet Med Austria/Wien Tierärztl Mschr 2008;95:56–63.

80. Cantatore M, Gobbetti M, Romussi S, et al. Medium term endoscopic assessment of the surgical outcome following laryngeal saccule resection in brachycephalic dogs. Vet Rec 2012;170:518.

81. Mehl ML, Kyles AE, Pypendop BH, et al. Outcome of laryngeal web resection with mucosal apposition for treatment of airway obstruction in dogs: 15 cases (1992–2006). J Am Vet Med Assoc 2008;233:738–42.

82. Matushek KJ, Bjorling DE. A mucosal flap technique for correction of laryngeal webbing. Results in four dogs. Vet Surg 1988;17:318–20.

83. Seim HB. Surgical management of brachycephalic syndrome. Proceedings North American Veterinary Conference. Orlando (FL): 2010.

84. Olivieri M, Voghera S, Fossum T. Video-assisted left partial arytenoidectomy by diode laser photoablation for treatment of canine laryngeal paralysis. Vet Surg 2009;38:439–44.

85. White RN. Surgical management of laryngeal collapse associated with brachycephalic airway obstruction syndrome in dogs. J Small Anim Pract 2012;53:44–50.

86. Hedlund CS. Brachycephalic syndrome. In: Bojrab MJ, Ellison GW, Slocum B, editors. Current techniques in small animal surgery. 4th edition. Baltimore (MD): Williams & Wilkins; 1998. p. 357–62.

87. Orsher R. Brachycephalic airway disease. In: Bojrab M, editor. Disease mechanisms in small animal surgery. 2nd edition. Philadelphia: Lea & Febiger; 1993. p. 369–70.

88. Harvey CE, O'Brien JA. Upper airway obstruction surgery 7: Tracheotomy in the dog and cat: analysis of 89 episodes in 79 animals. J Am Anim Hosp Assoc 1982; 18:563–6.

89. Nicholson I, Baines S. Complications associated with temporary tracheostomy tubes in 42 dogs (1998 to 2007). J Small Anim Pract 2012;53:108–14.

90. Senn D, Sigrist N, Fortere F, et al. Retrospective evaluation of postoperative nasotracheal tubes for oxygen supplementation in dogs following surgery for brachycephalic syndrome: 36 cases (2003-2007). J Vet Em Crit Care Med 2011;3:1–7.

91. Lorinson D, Bright RM, White RAS. Brachycephalic airway obstruction syndrome - a review of 118 cases. Canine Practice 1997;22:18–21.

92. Packer RMA, Hendricks A, Burn CC. Do dog owners perceive the clinical signs related to conformational inherited disorders as 'normal' for the breed? A potential constraint to improving canine welfare. Animal Welfare-The UFAW J 2012; 21:81.

Surgical Treatment of Laryngeal Paralysis

Eric Monnet, DVM, PhD

KEYWORDS

- Unilateral arytenoid lateralization • Arytenoidectomy • Ventral laryngotomy
- Permanent tracheostomy • Canine

KEY POINTS

- Unilateral arytenoid lateralization is the most commonly used technique to treat laryngeal paralysis.
- It is important not to overabduct the arytenoid cartilage during the unilateral lateralization to minimize exposure of the rima glottides.
- Dogs with laryngeal paralysis treated with unilateral lateralization have a good long-term prognosis.
- Idiopathic polyneuropathy is the most common cause of laryngeal paralysis in dogs.

INTRODUCTION

Laryngeal paralysis can be a manifestation of either a central neurologic lesion or a polyneuropathy. Congenital central neurologic lesions result in early signs (within months of birth) of laryngeal paralysis, while the clinical signs from acquired polyneuropathy occur in the later stages of life.[1]

Idiopathic polyneuropathy is the most common cause of laryngeal paralysis. Because the laryngeal recurrent laryngeal nerve is the longest nerve in the body, laryngeal paralysis is often the first clinical sign of a more generalized polyneuropathy. The recurrent laryngeal nerve is the only motor nerve of the larynx, and it innervates the cricoarytenoideus dorsalis muscle. During inspiration, the cricoarytenoideus dorsalis muscles abduct both arytenoid cartilages to reduce airway resistance and allow proper airflow. Therefore, dogs with laryngeal paralysis usually present with evidence of inspiratory difficulty.

Dogs with laryngeal paralysis should undergo complete physical examination, with focus on identifying neurologic deficits. The neurologic examination provides information on the severity and the stage of the polyneuropathy. Thoracic radiographs are

The author has nothing to disclose.
Department of Clinical Sciences, College of Veterinary Medicine and Biomedical Sciences, Colorado State University, 300 West Drake Road, Fort Collins, CO 80523, USA
E-mail address: Eric.Monnet@ColoState.EDU

important to evaluate lung parenchyma for aspiration pneumonia and also to detect evidence of megaesophagus. Megaesophagus and/or esophageal dysfunction may be seen as a progression of the polyneuropathy. Stanley and colleagues[1] demonstrated evidence of esophageal dysfunction in dogs with laryngeal paralysis, and recommended surgeons should perform a preoperative esophagram for dogs with laryngeal paralysis to help identify aspiration pneumonia risk. Concurrent esophageal disorders increase the risk of aspiration pneumonia after arytenoid lateralization surgery, which is designed to statically open the rima glottidis.

Definitive diagnosis of laryngeal paralysis is confirmed with laryngeal examination under heavy sedation with propofol as needed. Edema of the corniculate processes, laxity of the vocal cords, and lack of abduction of the arytenoid cartilages during inspiration are the criteria used to diagnose laryngeal paralysis. Doxapram hydrochloride, 1 mg/kg intravenously, can be administered intravenously during laryngeal examination to stimulate deeper breathing and augment abduction of the arytenoids.[2]

Dogs with laryngeal paralysis can present with an acute or chronic history suggesting upper airway obstruction. Clinicians evaluating dogs that present with acute airway compromise should obtain a more in-depth history from the owner, because there are often more subtle signs of airway disease such as a change in the bark, or exercise intolerance in the patient's past. Obvious signs associated with laryngeal paralysis are triggered during hot days, or during excitement or increased exercise. Dogs in an acute crisis often present in heat stroke and require emergency medical treatment. Sedation and oxygen therapy are appropriate for these dogs to help them calm down, and to help them ventilate. Administration of corticosteroids such as dexamethazone might be required in some cases refractory to standard medical care. If inspiratory dyspnea does not improve with these measures, general anesthesia with intubation or a temporary tracheostomy may be indicated. General anesthesia and intubation for 1 hour help provide more oxygen to the patient, improve ventilation, and help lower the body temperature. After 1 hour, the patient often is stable enough to be extubated. Temporary tracheostomy provides a bypass of the upper airway obstruction, and allows urgent transportation of the patient to an experienced surgeon for management. It should be noted, however, that patients requiring a temporary tracheostomy are at increased risk of aspiration pneumonia after surgical correction of laryngeal paralysis.[3] Acute upper airway obstruction can induce pulmonary edema. Fulminant pulmonary edema should be treated with oxygen supplementation, and an intravenously administered diuretic such as Furosemide, (2–4 mg/kg).

Dogs become candidates for surgical treatment when their quality of life is significantly affected by the laryngeal paralysis. If the owners are describing dramatic reduction in the level of exercise tolerance, or difficulty breathing with limited activity, surgery may be indicated.

SURGICAL THERAPY OPTIONS

Laryngeal paralysis requires surgical intervention to decrease airway resistance and improve airflow through the larynx. Several surgical techniques designed to open the rima glottidis have been reported, and each procedure has been shown to have differing outcomes. Partial arytenoidectomy with or without ventriculocordectomy, unilateral arytenoid lateralization, and permanent tracheostomy are the techniques most commonly used currently to treat laryngeal paralysis. Unilateral arytenoid lateralization is now recognized as the gold standard procedure to treat laryngeal paralysis. It has been shown to provide a consistently good outcome, and high owner satisfaction. Bilateral arytenoid lateralization is not recommended now, because it has been associated with a high risk of aspiration pneumonia and a high mortality rate.[3]

Partial Arytenoidectomy

Partial arytenoidectomy with ventriculocordectomy can be preformed via an oral approach or ventral laryngotomy. The goal of the procedure is to reduce airway resistance by removing tissue surrounding the rima glottidis.

Oral approach

After induction of general anesthesia, the dog is placed in sternal recumbency, and the mouth is held open with a mouth gag. The head of the dog is suspended and the tongue pulled forward. The soft palate is elevated with malleable retractors to visualize the larynx. Long instruments are recommended, because they do not interfere with visualization during the procedure. A cup biopsy forceps is used to remove portions of 1 corniculate process. Alternately, a scalpel blade can be used to partially resect the corniculate process. One vocal cord is also removed. In severe cases, the procedure can also be performed bilaterally. In this case, it is important to preserve the ventral portions of each vocal cord to help prevent scar tissue webbing across the rima glottidis. This procedure induces significant laryngeal inflammation in the early postoperative period, so the surgeon should be prepared to perform a temporary tracheostomy if necessary.

This technique results in 80% improvement in ventilation in the short term.[4] Long-term outcome was judged satisfactory in 90% of cases in 1 study.[4] A 60% 5-year survival rate has been reported.[3] Aspiration pneumonia, persistent cough, increased respiratory noise, and exercise intolerance have been reported in 6% to 53% of cases treated with arytenoidectomy.[5] Persistence of respiratory compromise has been reported in 18% of cases.[6]

Ventral approach

A ventral laryngotomy approach is the preferred approach for arytenoidectomy and ventriculocordectomy. With the oral approach, the laryngeal mucosal defect after vocal cordectomy is left to heal by second intension, which can generate significant scar tissue and eventually reobstruct the airway. Laryngeal webbing from scarring of cord remnants can occur in up to 14% of cases.[7] Mucosal defects from vocal cordectomy can be sutured closed via a ventral laryngotomy, and this allows primary healing of mucosa with less risk of mucosal webbing.[8]

The dog is placed in dorsal recumbency, and a ventral incision over the larynx is performed. Consider choosing a smaller-diameter endotracheal tube to reduce interference with visualization and suturing of the mucosal defects. The stenohyoideus muscles are separated and retracted. A #11 blade is used to incise the cricothyroid membrane and the thyroid cartilage on midline. The cranial part of the thyroid cartilage is left intact. Small Gelpi retractors are used to hold the larynx open to improve exposure. The corniculate and the cuneiform processes are resected with Metzenbaum scissors unilaterally or bilaterally.[9] The vocal cords are also resected. Mucosa of the laryngeal saccules is mobilized and sutured to the incised edges of the laryngeal mucosa with a 5-0 or 6-0 monofilament absorbable suture in a continuous pattern (**Fig. 1**). The larynx is then closed with a simple interrupted suture pattern. In a study on 88 dogs with laryngeal paralysis, satisfactory results were reported in 93% of the cases in the long term.[9] Aspiration pneumonia developed in 7% of the cases over the course of the study.[9]

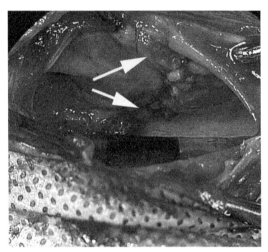

Fig. 1. A ventriculocordectomy has been performed and the mucosa from the laryngeal saccule has been sutured with a simple continuous suture pattern (*white arrows*) to cover the defect after resection of the vocal cords.

Unilateral Arytenoid Lateralization

Unilateral arytenoid lateralization is the surgical technique most commonly used to treat laryngeal paralysis. Originally, the procedure was described as being performed bilaterally, but this was associated with a high mortality rate from aspiration pneumonia.[3] The goal of the surgery is to abduct 1 arytenoid cartilage to open the rima glottidis and reduce airway resistance. If the abduction is too aggressive, the epiglottis cannot cover the rima glottides completely, and aspiration pneumonia may occur (**Fig. 2**). The goal is to optimize the abduction of 1 arytenoid cartilage without increasing the risk of aspiration pneumonia from overabduction.

The surgery can be performed with the dog in dorsal recumbency via a ventral midline approach, but most surgeons prefer a lateral approach currently. The ventral approach was mostly used when bilateral lateralization was performed, since both sides of the larynx can be readily accessed. However, now that unilateral lateralization is recommended, a lateral approach is most often used. The surgery can be performed on the left or the right side depending on surgeon preference. Right-handed surgeons usually prefer to conduct the surgery on the left side, because it is easier to forehand the needle when placing the cricoarytenoid suture.

After placing the dog in lateral recumbency, a roll of towels is placed under the neck of the dog to mound the larynx toward the surgeon. A skin incision is made ventral to the linguofacial vein over the thyroid cartilage region. After sharp dissection through the platysma muscle, the cranial border of the parotidus auricularis muscle is visible. The dissection continues cranial to this muscle through fat until the thyropharyngeal muscle is exposed. The dorsal border of the thyroid cartilage can then be palpated and rotated laterally. After incising the thyropharyngeal muscle along the dorsal border of the thyroid cartilage, a stay suture is passed through the thyroid cartilage (**Fig. 3**). This allows lateral rotation of the thyroid cartilage so the thyropharyngeal muscle can be excised caudally. The crico-thyroid joint is left intact and does not need to be disarticulated. The muscular process of the arytenoid cartilage can then be palpated. The cricoarytenoideus dorsalis muscle is then incised just caudal to the muscular process of the arytenoid process. The muscle can be rather normal

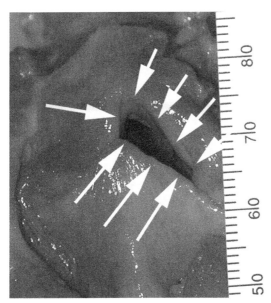

Fig. 2. A cadaveric image of the rima glottidis with overabduction of the arytenoid cartilage after unilateral lateralization. The white arrows indicate the surface area not covered by the epiglottis after lateralization of the right side. This opening may increase the risk of aspiration pneumonia.

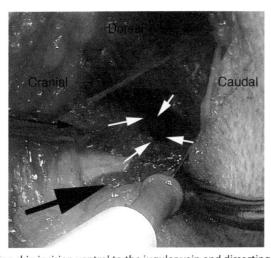

Fig. 3. After making skin incision ventral to the jugular vein and dissecting through the platisma muscle the thyropharyngeal muscle is exposed. In this image, the dorsal edge of the thyroid cartilage (*large black arrow*) has been retracted ventrally. The cricoarytenoideus dorsalis muscle has been transected and retracted cranially (*small black arrow*). The cricoarytenoid joint has been opened (*white arrows*). The author's preferred suture exit site in the cricoid cartilage is shown; the needle should exit just caudal to the cricoarytenoid joint (*black square*).

appearing or may appear very atrophied. The incision is performed with electrocoagulation to minimize bleeding from the edges of the muscle. The caudal aspect of the crico-arytenoid joint is incised. The incision should be wide enough to visualize the articular surface of the cricoid cartilage. A 2-0 prolonged absorbable or nonabsorbable monofilament suture is placed around the caudo-dorsal border of the cricoid cartilage to mimic the attachment of the cricoarytenoideus dorsalis muscle. A thumb forceps can be placed behind the caudal border of the cricoid cartilage to push down on the endotracheal tube to prevent incorporating it in this needle bite. It is important not to place the suture too dorsal to avoid damaging the esophagus. The author prefers to drive the needle cranio-ventrally through the cricoid cartilage, exiting just caudal to the joint capsule of the crico-arytenoid joint. The suture is placed through the muscular process of the arytenoid cartilage. The suture is then tied to abduct the arytenoid cartilage. Because the suture exits along the caudal border of the crico-arytenoid joint, it helps limit the risk of overabduction of the arytenoid cartilage during suture tensioning. The thyropharyngeal muscle is then closed with 4-0 absorbable monofilament in simple continuous pattern. Bupivacaine (1 mg/kg) is applied in the surgical field as a line or splash block. Subcutaneous tissue and skin are closed in a routine fashion.

Instead of placing the suture around the cricoid cartilage as described previously, some surgeons instead place the suture through the thyroid cartilage.[10] It is felt that placement in this fashion pulls the arytenoid cartilage in more a lateral direction. It has been shown to be a faster procedure than when the suture is placed around the cricoid cartilage.[11] However, placement of the suture through the thyroid cartilage has been shown to result in less enlargement of surface area of the rima glottidis compared with the cricoid cartilage suture technique.[11] Placement of 2 lateralization sutures, one through the thyroid cartilage and one through the cricoid, has been evaluated.[12] A randomized clinical trial demonstrated that there is no benefit in placing 2 sutures, because doing so does not improve the surface area of the rima glottidis. Furthermore, placing 2 sutures through the small muscular process may increase the risk of fracture if the needle is not carefully positioned. It is the author's preference to place just 1 suture around the cricoid cartilage, because it reproduces more closely the anatomy of the cricoarytenoideus dorsalis muscle; additionally, the amount of the abduction of the arytenoid cartilage can be better controlled. The thyroarytenoid suture has a tendency to induce a lateral displacement instead of a caudolateral displacement of the arytenoid cartilage.

Placement of the suture in the muscular process of the arytenoid cartilage can result in fracturing of the cartilage. Therefore, it is important to aim for the thickest part of the muscular process when placing the needle. If the arytenoid cartilage fractures, it is generally recommended to abandon the original approach, and perform the procedure on the other side. However, in the author's experience, the surgery can be salvaged by repairing the cartilage fracture with a mattress suture. Double-armed 3-0 monofilament nonabsorbable suture is chosen for this repair. After placing 1 arm of the suture around the caudo-dorsal border of the cricoid cartilage, it will then be possible to place both arms in the muscular process of the arytenoid cartilage. A Dacron pledget can be used to reinforce the suture and prevent tearing through the muscular process cartilage.

The amount of tension or abduction of the arytenoid cartilage necessary to allow adequate ventilation but without creating an incompetent seal of the rima glottidis has been the subject of several recent investigations. All the techniques used to treat laryngeal paralysis have been shown to increase the surface area of the rima glottidis.[13] The ideal surface area of rima glottidis to sufficiently reduce airway resistance is still not known. Because the airway resistance is inversely related to the radius to the fourth power, it is probably not necessary to abduct the arytenoid cartilage fully to achieve a significant reduction of airway resistance and adequate clinical improvement.[14] It has been hypothesized that overabduction of the arytenoid cartilage can increase the risk of aspiration pneumonia, because the epiglottis cannot completely cover the rima glottidis.[15] Intraoperative visualization of the amount of abduction achieved during surgery has been advocated.[16] It requires extubation of the patient during the procedure, and visualization of the larynx with a laryngoscope or endoscope. When an endoscope is used, the amount of abduction can be adjusted in real time by the surgeon while viewing the monitor. The amount of tension placed on the suture has been shown to affect the surface area of the rima glottidis.[15] However, the amount of suture tension necessary to adequately abduct the arytenoid cartilage is subjective. A tensiometer has been used in 1 study to help determine the optimal suture tension, but this is not very practical in a clinical situation.[17] Gauthier and Monnet[18] demonstrated the optimal placement of the needle during cricoarytenoid suturing was caudal to the crico-arytenoid joint in a canine cadaveric study. This needle exit landmark in the cricoid cartilage resulted in significant reduction of airway resistance during the inspiration phase while not creating gaps between the rima glottides and epiglottis when the epiglottis was closed. Placement of the cricoarytenoid suture in this fashion using this anatomic landmark helps eliminate the subjective nature of the tension on the suture.[14] The suture exiting the cricoid cartilage caudal to the joint capsule will limit excessive abduction of the arytenoid cartilage. The author believes this technique limits the tension on the suture in the arytenoid muscular process, and this might reduce the risk of cartilage fracture or tearing out of the suture and failure of the procedure.

Bilateral arytenoid lateralization has been combined with vocal fold excision in 67 dogs with laryngeal paralysis.[19] Nineteen dogs had recurrence of the clinical signs caused by narrowing of the rima glottides, and 3 dogs developed aspiration pneumonia. A partial arytenoidectomy had to be performed to resolve the narrowing of the larynx in the dogs with rima glottides narrowing.

In an effort to minimize soft tissue trauma, and preserve the cricopharyngeal muscle and the intrinsic nerve branches to the larynx, a less invasive approach for arytenoid lateralization has been described.[20] The approach was developed to minimize dysfunction of the thyropharyngeal and cricopharyngeal muscles that could result in dysphagia and aspiration pneumonia. The rate of aspiration pneumonia was 18% in this study, which is similar to rates using the standard unilateral lateralization technique.[3,20] Bahr and colleagues[21] compared the outcome of dogs with laryngeal paralysis treated with ventriculocordectomy or unilateral lateralization. Dogs with ventriculocordectomy had more long-term complications associated with chronic respiratory distress, and required more surgical revisions than the dogs treated with unilateral lateralization.[21] Therefore, unilateral lateralization using 1 suture is considered the most commonly performed procedure for treatment of laryngeal paralysis currently.

Complications associated with unilateral lateralization include seroma, infection, aspiration pneumonia, persistent coughing, and recurrence of clinical signs. Recurrence of clinical signs usually results from either fracture of the arytenoid cartilage or tear-out of the suture following surgery. The risk of lateralization failure is highest within the first 2 to 3 weeks after surgery. There is no well-established recommendation about feeding habits after unilateral arytenoid lateralization. Dogs can be fed their regular diet after surgery.

Aspiration pneumonia occurs after unilateral lateralization in 8% to 21% of the cases reported to date.[22] Likely, the placement of the suture and the amount of abduction influence the risk of pneumonia following surgery.[15] Other risk factors for development of aspiration pneumonia include megaesophagus before or after surgery, temporary tracheostomy, and preoperative pneumonia.[3] Dogs with laryngeal paralysis have an idiopathic polyneuropathy that can induce esophageal dysfunction.[1] Progression of generalized polyneuropathy can occur within 1 year after laryngeal repair, and this has been shown to affect long-term prognosis.[1] However, progression of the poly-neuropathy may be variable between studies. In 1 study of 140 dogs treated for laryngeal paralysis with unilateral cricoarytenoid lateralization, the 5-year survival rate was 70%.[3]

Permanent Tracheostomy

Permanent tracheostomy is a procedure reserved for dogs with concurrent megaeso-phagus and signs of regurgitation. This procedure allows adequate ventilation, since it completely bypasses the upper airway obstruction.

Surgical technique

The patient is placed in dorsal recumbency. A longitudinal skin incision is performed caudal to the larynx over the trachea. After the dissection between the sternohyoideus muscles, the trachea is exposed. The sternohydeus muscle can be sutured dorsal to the trachea to gain better exposure of the trachea and reduce tension on the tracheal mucosa skin closure. The tracheal window is created with a length of 3 to 4 tracheal rings and a width one-third the size of the tracheal diameter. The segment of the tracheal cartilage rings should be removed without damaging the underlying tracheal mucosa. The tracheal mucosa is then incised and sutured to the skin with a 4-0 mono-filament nonabsorbable suture. It is important to achieve a good apposition of the skin with the tracheal mucosa to prevent stricture formation. A simple interrupted suture pattern is often chosen to provide the best mucosal–skin apposition.

Complications

Complications associated with permanent tracheostomy include chronic respiratory infection, inhalation of foreign materials, aspiration of water during bathing or swim-ming, and chronic mucus discharge from the tracheostomy.

SUMMARY

Dogs with laryngeal paralysis showing significant signs of respiratory compromise are surgical candidates. The unilateral lateralization seems to provide the most predict-able long-term outcome. Surgery should be expected to dramatically improve quality of life in the long term. Dogs are at risk of aspiration pneumonia for the rest of their life.

REFERENCES

1. Stanley BJ, Hauptman JG, Fritz MC, et al. Esophageal dysfunction in dogs with idiopathic laryngeal paralysis: a controlled cohort study. Vet Surg 2010;39:139–49.
2. Tobias KM, Jackson AM, Harvey RC. Effects of doxapram HCl on laryngeal func-tion of normal dogs and dogs with naturally occurring laryngeal paralysis. Vet Anaesth Analg 2004;31:258–63.
3. MacPhail CM, Monnet E. Outcome of and postoperative complications in dogs undergoing surgical treatment of laryngeal paralysis: 140 cases (1985-1998). J Am Vet Med Assoc 2001;218:1949–56.
4. Holt D, Harvey C. Idiopathic laryngeal paralysis—results of treatment by bilateral vocal fold resection in 40 dogs. J Am Anim Hosp Assoc 1994;30:389–95.

5. Harvey CE. Upper airway obstruction surgery. 4. Partial laryngectomy in brachy-cephalic dogs. J Am Anim Hosp Assoc 1982;18:548–50.
6. Ross JT, Matthiesen DT, Noone KE, et al. Complications and long-term results after partial laryngectomy for the treatment of idiopathic laryngeal paralysis in 45 dogs. Vet Surg 1991;20:169–73.
7. Holt D, Harvey C. Glottic stenosis secondary to vocal fold resection—results of scar removal and corticosteroid treatment in 9 dogs. J Am Anim Hosp Assoc 1994;30:396–400.
8. Mehl ML, Kyles AE, Pypendop BH, et al. Outcome of laryngeal web resection with mucosal apposition for treatment of airway obstruction in dogs: 15 cases (1992–2006). J Am Vet Med Assoc 2008;233:738–42.
9. Zikes C, McCarthy T. Bilateral ventriculocordectomy via ventral laryngotomy for idiopathic laryngeal paralysis in 88 dogs. J Am Anim Hosp Assoc 2012;48:234–44.
10. White RAS. Unilateral aytenoid lateralisation: an assessment of technique and long term results in 62 dogs with laryngeal paralysis. J Small Anim Pract 1989;30:543–9.
11. Griffiths LG, Sullivan M, Reid SW. A comparison of the effects of unilateral thyro-arytenoid lateralization versus cricoarytenoid laryngoplasty on the area of the rima glottidis and clinical outcome in dogs with laryngeal paralysis. Vet Surg 2001;30:359–65.
12. Demetriou JL, Kirby BM. The effect of two modifications of unilateral arytenoid lateralization on rima glottidis area in dogs. Vet Surg 2003;32:62–8.
13. Harvey CE. Partial laryngectomy in the dog. 2. Immediate increase in glottic area obtained compared with other laryngeal procedures. Vet Surg 1983;12:197–201.
14. Greenberg MJ, Bureau S, Monnet E. Effects of suture tension during unilateral cricoarytenoid lateralization on canine laryngeal resistance in vitro. Vet Surg 2007;36:526–32.
15. Bureau S, Monnet E. Effects of suture tension and surgical approach during unilateral arytenoid lateralization on the rima glottidis in the canine larynx. Vet Surg 2002;31:589–95.
16. Weinstein J, Weisman D. Intraoperative evaluation of the larynx following unilateral arytenoid lateralization for acquired idiopathic laryngeal paralysis in dogs. J Am Anim Hosp Assoc 2010;46:241–8.
17. Wignall JR, Baines SJ. Effects of unilateral arytenoid lateralization technique and suture tension on airway pressure in the larynx of canine cadavers. Am J Vet Res 2012;73:917–24.
18. Gauthier CM, Monnet E. In vitro evaluation of anatomic landmarks for the placement of suture to achieve effective arytenoid cartilage abduction by means of unilateral cricoarytenoid lateralization in dogs. Am J Vet Res 2014;75:602–6.
19. Schofield DM, Norris J, Sadanaga KK. Bilateral thyroarytenoid cartilage lateralization and vocal fold excision with mucosoplasty for treatment of idiopathic laryngeal paralysis: 67 dogs (1998-2005). Vet Surg 2007;36:519–25.
20. von Pfeil DJ, Edwards MR, Dejardin LM. Less invasive unilateral arytenoid lateralization: a modified technique for treatment of idiopathic laryngeal paralysis in dogs: technique description and outcome. Vet Surg 2014;43:704–11.
21. Bahr KL, Howe L, Jessen C, et al. Outcome of 45 dogs with laryngeal paralysis treated by unilateral arytenoid lateralization or bilateral ventriculocordectomy. J Am Anim Hosp Assoc 2014;50:264–72.
22. White RAS. Arytenoid lateralization:an assessment of technique, complications and long-term results in 62 dogs with laryngeal paralysis. Vet Surg 1989;18:72.

Surgical Approaches to the Nasal Cavity and Sinuses

Alyssa Marie Weeden, DVM, Daniel Alvin Degner, DVM*

KEYWORDS

- Nasal cavity • Sinuses • Turbinates • CT scan • Rhinotomy • Mucoperiosteum
- Neoplasia

KEY POINTS

- CT scan of the head is the best diagnostic for initial evaluation of nasal cavity diseases.
- Most nasal cavity tumors in dogs are locally invasive and late to metastasize.
- Nasal cavity tumors are largely treated with radiation; however, adjunctive surgery is beneficial in some patients.
- The ventral approach to the nasal cavity provides an excellent avenue to the nasal cavity and nasopharygeal lesions.

The nasal cavity is the first portion of the respiratory tract and begins with the external nares and ends with the nasal conchae. The nasopharynx extends from the conchae to the intrapharyngeal ostium, which is just cranial to the larynx.

The paranasal or frontal sinuses extend very far caudally on the head of most canine breeds. The exception lies in canine breeds classified as brachycephalics, such as Boston terrier, Bulldogs, Pugs, Shih Tzus, Boxers, and Pekinese, which have very compact frontal sinuses and do not extend far caudally on the head (**Fig. 1**). There are three compartments of the frontal sinuses: (1) the large caudal, (2) smaller rostral, and (3) medial compartments. The latter drain via an ostia into the caudodorsal nasal cavity. The floor of the frontal sinuses extends over the olfactory and rostral part of the frontal lobes of the brain. For this important reason one must avoid penetration of this portion of the sinuses with curettes, drills, and other instruments.

Maxillary sinuses are small and consequential when abscessation of caudal maxillary premolar teeth is present. The maxillary sinus or recess is a lateral diverticulum of the nasal cavity and has its opening at the level of the rostral roots of the fourth upper premolar tooth (**Fig. 2**).

The authors have nothing to disclose.
Animal Surgical Center of Michigan, 5045 Miller Road, Flint, MI 48507, USA
* Corresponding author.
E-mail address: ddegner@comcast.net

Vet Clin Small Anim 46 (2016) 719–733
http://dx.doi.org/10.1016/j.cvsm.2016.02.004
0195-5616/16/$ – see front matter
vetsmall.theclinics.com

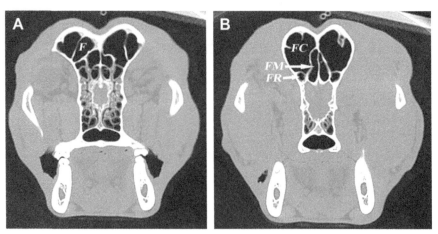

Fig. 1. Rottweiler, 3-year-old female spayed. (*A*) Transverse plane computed tomography (CT) images of normal frontal sinus anatomy. The frontal sinus region is denoted by the letter F. (*B*) The frontal sinus region is denoted by FC, FR, and FM, which refer to the caudal, rostral, and medial compartments. **Fig. 1**A is more rostral compared with **Fig. 1**B.

The nasal cavity is separated along the midline sagittal plane by a membranous, osseous, and cartilaginous nasal septum. The conchae, also known as turbinates, are scrolled bones of the nasal cavity that purify and humidify inspired air (**Fig 3**). The dorsal, ventral, and ethmoidal conchae fill most of the nasal cavity. The dorsal and ventral conchae attach on the ethmoid, nasal, and maxillary bones. The ethmoidal

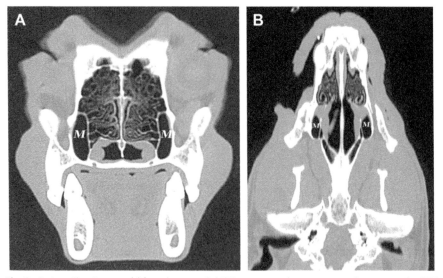

Fig. 2. Rottweiler, 3-year-old female spayed. (*A*) Transverse plane computed tomography (CT) image of normal canine maxillary sinus anatomy. (*B*) Dorsal coronal plane CT image of normal canine maxillary sinus anatomy. The maxillary sinus region is denoted by the letter M.

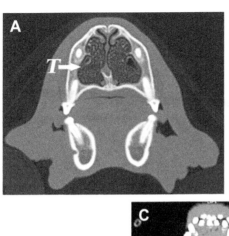
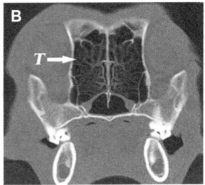
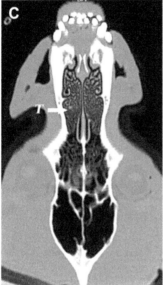

Fig. 3. (*A, B*) Rottweiler, 3-year-old male intact. Normal canine turbinate anatomy. (*C*) Rottweiler, 5-year-old female spayed. Dorsal coronal plane computed tomography (CT) image of normal canine anatomy is denoted by the letter T for turbinates.

conchae attach only to the ethmoid bones, which form the rostral aspect of the cranial vault. The medial canthus of the eye approximates the level of the ethmoidal conchae. An extremely vascular mucosal lining covers the nasal turbinates. Therefore, significant hemorrhage is typically experienced during turbinate ablation surgery or turbinate biopsy procedures.

The blood supply of the nasal cavity comes primarily from the maxillary artery, which is an extension of the external carotid. The maxillary artery branches into the infraorbital artery, which perfuses the tissues external to the nasal cavity and the sphenopalatine and major palatine arteries, which perfuse the palate and the conchae of the nasal cavity. The major palatine artery provides blood supply to most of the hard palate and the minor palatine artery perfuses the caudal aspect of the hard palate. The ethmoidal conchae are also perfused by the internal ethmoidal arteries, which penetrate through the rostral aspect of the cranial vault by passage through the cribiform plate. Venous drainage parallels the arterial supply; however, externally venous drainage is via branches of the facial vein.

The trigeminal nerve splits into three separate branches: (1) the ophthalmic, (2) maxillary, and (3) mandibular divisions. The maxillary nerve parallels the maxillary artery as described previously. Further branching of the maxillary nerve provides innervation of the nasal mucosa, roots of maxillary teeth, and glands. The facial nerve, which divides into several branches, is primarily responsible for motor innervation of all superficial muscles of the head and some muscles of the neck.

The maxillary, premaxillary, nasal, frontal, sphenoid, and palatine bones provide the primary structure of the nasal cavity.[1,2]

BIOPSY OF SINONASAL LESIONS

Lesions within the nasal cavity are easily accessed via the nares. Lesions are visualized with a rigid endoscope followed by biopsies obtained with endoscopic forceps that are run in an operating channel of the telescope cannula. Only small biopsy specimens can be obtained with this method and there is a risk that nondiagnostic samples may be obtained. As a result, large tissue samples can be obtained by blindly grasping tissue samples with cup biopsy forceps. The depth to which the forceps should be inserted into the nasal cavity is based on computed tomography (CT) imagery. If the tumor has eroded through the dorsal or lateral wall of the nasal cavity, a small skin incision can be made over the area of interest and a tissue sample collected. If the tumor is located in the frontal sinuses and only marginally extending into the nasal cavity, then the frontal sinus can be trephinated and cup biopsy forceps used to collect tissue samples. If the tumor is in the caudal nasal cavity, samples may be collected with the aid of a flexible endoscope that is retroflexed up the nasopharynx.

SURGICAL TREATMENT OF LESIONS WITHIN THE NASAL CAVITY AND FRONTAL SINUSES

Most tumors of the nasal cavity are locally invasive and malignant in dogs and cats (**Fig. 4**A–C).[3,4] Carcinomas including adenocarcinoma and squamous cell carcinomas and sarcomas including chondrosarcoma, fibrosarcoma, osteosarcoma, and undifferentiated sarcoma comprise most nasal tumors.[5] Of these, nasal cavity adenocarcinoma is by far the most common tumor. Some lesions of the nasal and frontal sinuses may be amended with surgical modalities. Previously, surgical removal or debulking of all nasal tumors and adjunctive radiation therapy was the treatment of choice.[6] Megavoltage radiation (linear accelerator or cobalt source) therapy then became the mainstay for treatment of nasal tumors without surgery.[5,7] More recently, radiation therapy followed up by surgical excision of the contents of the nasal cavity has been shown to increase the disease-free interval for dogs having certain nasal tumors.[8] The efficacy of chemotherapeutic agents used as a single curative treatment option is infrequently selected and therefore the true role of this treatment modality is undetermined.[5] Other lesions that necessitate surgical exploration of the nasal cavity include foreign bodies and *Cuterebra* infestation that cannot be safely removed using endoscopic techniques.[9]

Fungal disease of the nasal cavity and sinuses can also result in clinical signs similar to nasal cavity neoplasia. Unique to fungal rhinitis is depigmentation of the nasal planum caused by toxins from the fungus. Fungal organisms, such as *Aspergillus* spp, uncommonly *Penicillium* spp, or rarely *Rhinosporidium* spp, commonly destroy the nasal turbinates, leaving a void in the nasal cavity (**Fig. 4**D). Treatment involves topical

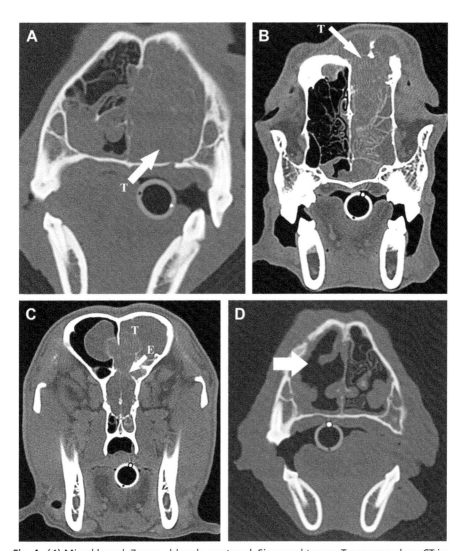

Fig. 4. (A) Mixed breed, 7-year-old male neutered. Sinonasal tumor. Transverse plane CT image reconstructed in bone. The right nasal cavity is almost completely filled with a soft tissue mass (*arrow*) and there is the absence of nasal turbinates. The patient was diagnosed with a locally invasive nasal adenocarcinoma. (B) Golden retriever, 9-year-old female spayed. Sinonasal tumor. Transverse plane CT image. The right nasal cavity is completely filled with a soft tissue opacity. (C) There is extension into the rostral brain and frontal sinus indicated by the *arrow* denoting region of extension. No further diagnostics were pursued to determine diagnosis. (D) Mixed breed, 5-year-old female spayed. Fungal rhinitis. Bilateral destruction of nasal turbinates denoted by the *arrow* and turbinate destruction is worse on the left compared with the right. Further diagnostics determined *Aspergillosis* to be the causative agent.

infusion of clotrimazole solution followed by clotrimazole cream into small trephination holes made in each frontal sinus. A single midline skin incision is centered over the frontal sinus (based on CT scan). The skin is moved over to the center of the left frontal sinus (in normocephalic dogs this is at the level of the lateral orbital ligament). A

2.7-mm drill bit is placed in a drill and choked up in the chuck so that about 5 mm is extending from the end of a 2.7-mm drill sleeve, thus minimizing the risk of deep penetration into the brain. The process is repeated on the right frontal sinus. An 8F red rubber catheter (with the end cut off) is inserted into the left trephination hole and the sinonasal cavity is flushed; the process is repeated on the right side. Then, clotrimazole solution is instilled into each side followed by clotrimazole cream. Most dogs respond well to one treatment, yet for those that do not respond completely, a second treatment is needed.

Lesions in the area of the choanae and the nasopharynx include infiltrative tumors (eg, adenocarcinoma, chondrosarcoma, squamous cell carcinoma, lymphoma), nasopharyngeal polyps, foreign bodies, nasopharyngeal strictures, and obstructive aberrant turbinates as seen in brachycephalic breeds. Nasal cavity polyps may be exposed and retrieved by cranial retraction of the soft palate. For those more rostrally located, a midline ventral approach through the rostral soft palate and caudal hard palate generally provides excellent access (**Fig. 5**). Aggressive debridement of this area may result in stricture of the area after healing takes place. Foreign bodies, if not retrievable with flexible endoscopy, may be retrieved using a similar approach. Nasopharyngeal strictures are more commonly treated with minimally invasive techniques using endoscopic bougienage and potentially placement of a stent. (See Berent AC: Diagnosis and Management of Nasopharyngeal Stenosis, in this issue.) Obstructive

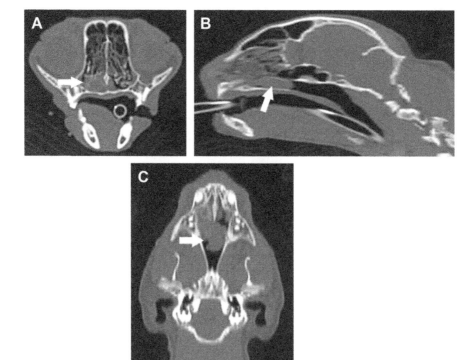

Fig. 5. Domestic medium hair, 15-year-old female spayed. CT images reveal a ventral nasal cavity polyp (*arrow*) on the right side. Transverse image (*A*), sagittal image (*B*), and a dorsal plane image (*C*). Histopathology confirmed inflammatory polyp following removal.

nasopharyngeal turbinates, as seen in brachycephalics, are usually removed endo-scopically with laser; however, a ventral approach to the affected area is also used for surgical removal.

PATIENT PREPARATION FOR NASAL SURGERY

A complete physical examination should be completed on each patient before diag-nostic testing to rule out other systemic diseases, which may increase surgical morbidity and mortality. The comprehensive preoperative work-up should consist of analyses including a complete blood cell count, serum biochemical profile, urinalysis, coagulation profile (prothrombin time/partial thromboplastin time and activated clot-ting time [ACT]), systemic blood pressure, electrocardiogram, oximetry, and von Wil-lebrand factor level in suspect breeds. Imaging, comprised of numerous modalities, should also be incorporated to determine the extent of disease and appropriate sur-gical planning. Three-view (left lateral, right lateral, and ventrodorsal) thoracic radio-graphs or chest CT scan should be acquired to evaluate the patient when neoplasia is a primary differential diagnosis. CT is an excellent modality to evaluate the extent and nature of nasal diseases and helps the surgeon develop a surgical plan for the pa-tient. MRI is also an excellent modality beneficial in the diagnosis of nasal tumors, fungal disease, and potentially foreign bodies. CT scan and MRI perform similarly in the identification of feline and canine intranasal neoplasia detection.[10] The decision on what type of advanced imaging is at the discretion of the surgeon. Nasal radio-graphs have a low diagnostic yield to define the type or extent of nasal disease and are usually of no value for surgical decision-making.

Hydration status, assessed by physical examination and diagnostic testing, aids in determining if intravenous fluid therapy is essential before surgery in such cases where the patient has become debilitated from the nasal disease. Most patients, however, do not have this complicating factor.

Although nasal cavity surgery is associated with brisk, profuse hemorrhage, mini-mizing blood loss is essential. During the procedure, bleeding is controlled by the use of electrocoagulation, digital pressure, and iced saline spiked with epinephrine (1:100,000).[11,12] The best method of minimizing nasal cavity hemorrhage is speed of surgery; after the turbinates and tumor have been extirpated, the hemorrhage slows down dramatically and the cavity can be packed with sterile saline-soaked sponges if needed. Another method to implement is temporary carotid occlusion before sur-gery, which reduces blood loss during surgery of the nasal cavity and can be safely used over a period of 2 to 3 hours.[12,13] When the common carotid arteries are occluded, the brain is still perfused adequately by the basilar artery via the vertebral artery. This procedure is not recommended in cats because the circulatory system to the brain may depend on the common carotid arteries and the basilar system may be underdeveloped. Hypotension during surgery may also compound poor brain perfusion with carotid occlusion in this species, which results in profound postopera-tive neurologic signs.

To perform temporary carotid artery occlusion, a midline incision is made over the ventral cervical region from the larynx to the manubrium. The platysma muscle is incised. The sternohyoid muscles are separated on the midline of the neck by blunt and sharp dissection. Critical structures that must not be injured during the approach include the trachea and recurrent laryngeal nerves, which run along the dorsolateral aspect of the trachea; esophagus (which is on the left dorsolateral aspect of the tra-chea); and the vagosympathetic trunks. To safely preserve the vagosympathetic trunks, each carotid sheath is incised with fine scissors and the nerve is separated from the common carotid artery. The common carotid arteries can be occluded with a Rummel tourniquet consisting of a strand of umbilical tape. The tape is threaded through a 3-inch section of a red rubber catheter of appropriate diameter. Alternatively, the arteries can be occluded with appropriate-sized vascular clamps, such as microvascular or bulldog clamps.[9,11,13–15] Once the nasal cavity procedure is completed, the vascular clamps are removed and the neck wound is closed. Most surgeons do not use carotid occlusion during nasal surgery, and it is only used for select cases (eg, expected more severe hemorrhage, patient with marginal anemia, brain case invasion, and surgical time may be increased because of more delicate surgery).[13]

SURGICAL APPROACHES

There are four surgical approaches to expose the nasal cavity and sinuses. The dorsal approach is selected most frequently to access the nasal cavity and frontal sinuses. The ventral approach is the preferred method to access the nasal cavity and nasopharyngeal region. The combined rostrolateral rhinotomy approach, although uncommonly used, allows access to the rostral nasal septal region. The fourth approach provides visualization of the caudal pharyngeal region.

Dorsal Approach

The dorsal approach is useful to access the entire nasal cavity and the frontal sinuses. This approach can be used for most diseases of the nasal cavity except for lesions located within the nasopharynx (**Fig. 6**). The patient is placed in ventral recumbency and the skin aseptically prepared. A midline skin incision is made with a number 10 blade from the caudal extent of the sinuses to a point just caudal to the nasal planum followed by the subcutaneous layer. Care is taken especially at the rostral extent of the incision to avoid veins that encroach along the midline. Any superficial bleeding is arrested with electrocoagulation. The periosteum is incised and elevated by using a periosteal elevator from the midline to the lateral aspect of the frontal sinuses and the maxillary bones. Gelpi retractors or stay sutures are used to aid in direct visualization of the underlying bone. To approach the nasal cavity, either a "lid" osteotomy is made or the bone is removed. The "lid" osteotomy is performed by making a beveled osteotomy around the dorsal aspect of the nasal cavity and frontal sinus (if these also need to be explored) with a sagittal saw and a thin kerf saw blade. Beveling of the osteotomy helps to minimize the risk of the lid falling into the nasal cavity and frontal sinuses during closure of the dorsal rhinotomy. If the bone is healthy, it can be saved in sterile saline-soaked sponges, and replaced when closure is begun. At the conclusion of the nasal surgery, 1-mm holes are drilled in the border of the rostral, middle, and caudal regions of the bony lid and the surrounding bone and the lid is then secured in place with twisted 26-gauge stainless steel wire. Periosteum is then sutured over the bony lid using a simple interrupted pattern of 4–0 polydioxanone suture (PDS). The subcutaneous layer is closed followed by the skin with either external sutures or an intradermal pattern.

More commonly, dorsal rhinotomy is performed by removing a window of bone over the dorsal bridge of the nose and frontal sinuses using one of two techniques. A pneumatic drill with a 2- to 4-mm burr is used to remove the bone from the proposed rhinotomy site. The area should be liberally lavaged with cold sterile saline during the procedure to minimize the risk of thermal necrosis of the adjacent bone. Alternatively, a large intramedullary pin may be inserted through the nasal bone and then a rongeur is used to remove bone from the dorsal nasal cavity and frontal sinuses. It is essential

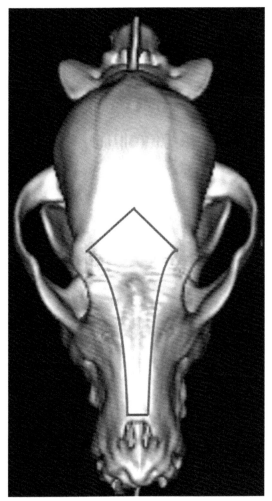

Fig. 6. Canine skull. Three-dimensional CT reconstruction. Dorsal rhinosinusotomy. The *red line* illustrates the limits of the osteotomy, lid or excisional.

to avoid extending the rhinotomy window over the lateral aspect of the bridge of the nose because this results in facial deformity.

Closure of the dorsal rhinotomy involves suturing the periosteum over the midline with an interrupted pattern using 4–0 PDS. The subcutaneous layer and skin are closed routinely with either external sutures or an intradermal pattern.[10]

Ventral Approach

The ventral approach is useful to access the nasal cavity and nasopharyngeal region. The frontal sinuses, however, cannot be explored using this approach. The advantage to this approach is that the complication of subcutaneous emphysema does not occur as it does with a dorsal approach. An uncommon complication that may occur is a persistent oronasal fistula, which may result in chronic infection of the nasal cavity and subsequent nasal discharge. The patient is placed in dorsal recumbency and the oral cavity rinsed with dilute chlorhexidine gluconate (1:40) or povidone-iodine solution (1:100). To perform this approach, an incision is made in the mucoperiosteum along the midline of the hard palate with a number 15 or 11 blade. A periosteal elevator is used to elevate the tissues off the palatine bone. Stay sutures instead of traumatic gelpi retractors can be placed in the tissues on either side of midline to allow for better visualization of the underlying bone. Care is taken to avoid lacerating the caudal and rostral major palatine vessels as they exit the rostral, and caudal palatine foramina located near medial to the fourth upper premolar teeth. After the mucoperiosteum has been elevated adequately, the bone is removed using a pneumatic drill and burr (**Fig. 7**). The intranasal procedure is therefore performed. Closure of the mucoperiosteum is completed in one or two layers using prolonged absorbable suture, such as 4–0 Biosyn or PDS, in a simple continuous or interrupted pattern.[11–14]

Combined Rostrolateral Nasal Approach

Tumors affecting the rostral nasal septum may be removed using a rostral approach. Careful selection of acceptable cases for this technique is performed with the evaluation of a CT or MRI study. This technique is limited to small (<1 cm) squamous cell carcinomas or other local or benign tumors affecting the rostral septum. The nasal planum is elevated as a dorsally-based U-shaped flap; the flap generally is about 5 mm thick to minimize the risk of penetrating into the tumor. A lateral rhinotomy incision is then made on the ipsilateral side of the mass by extending a skin incision from the angle of the rhinarium to the nasomaxillary notch with subsequent transection of the maxillary cartilage between the dorsal and ventral parietal cartilages. The tumor is then exposed and the affected septal resection is performed. This area is left to heal by second intension. The lateral rhinotomy is closed in three layers (mucosal/cartilage, submucosal, and skin); the U-shaped rostral flap is closed with simple interrupted sutures ventrally.[16,17]

Nasopharyngeal Approach

This intraoral approach is used for foreign bodies and surgical resection of masses located in the nasopharyngeal region, dorsal to the soft palate. The approach is made with the patient in ventral recumbency and the mouth fully open with a mouth gag. Alternatively, if additional exposure to the pharyngeal region is needed, the mandibular symphysis may be separated with an osteotome or sagittal saw and soft tissues on the lateral aspect of the tongue may be incised; in the author's experience, this approach is uncommonly needed.[11,18] A full-thickness incision is made in the soft palate from the caudal aspect of the hard palate to a point just rostral to the end of the soft palate. Leaving the terminal part of the soft palate intact reduces the incidence of dehiscence of the incision during the healing phase. The incised edges of the palate are retracted open with stay sutures placed on each side of the incision. Closure of the incision is performed with absorbable sutures, such as 4–0 to 5–0 PDS or Monocryl in an interrupted pattern. If possible a three-layer closure is performed: nasopharyngeal mucosal layer is closed first, then the muscle layer, and finally the oral mucosal layer. To reduce irritation in the oral cavity, knots that are buried may be used. Meticulous closure is essential to overcome incisional tension exerted by the tensor palatine muscles.[9,10]

SURGICAL EXTIRPATION OF NASAL TUMORS AND DISEASED TURBINATES

A variety of techniques are used to ablate the contents of the nasal cavity. Rongeurs are typically useful to grasp and tear the turbinates and associated tumor from the nasal cavity. This should be done expediently because hemorrhage tends to be fairly brisk during this part of the procedure. Care must be taken because the ethmoidal turbinates are removed. This area of the cranium is thin and inadvertent penetration into the brain may occur with aggressive surgical technique. The ethmoid turbinates normally are gray color compared with the typical red color of the nasal turbinates. Fairly large palatine vessels located on the caudolateral aspect of the floor of the nasal cavity can also be a source of significant hemorrhage and should be avoided. After the nasal turbinates have been removed, the rostral aspect of the nasal cavity must be evaluated to ensure that nares are patent. Transection of the rostral limit of the turbinates and septum, which are cartilaginous, with a number 11 scalpel blade ensures that no tissue is occluding the rostral respiratory passage. The opening into the nasopharynx, the conchae, must also be evaluated to ensure that no residual tumor or turbinate tissue is occluding this region. If residual tumor or turbinate tissue is found to be blocking this region, delicate retrieval by means of curved hemostatic forceps is necessary. For the most part, surgeons have abandoned using surgery as a primary role in the treatment of malignant nasal tumors and radiation therapy is the preferred treatment. Fibrosarcoma of the nasal cavity is optimally treated both with radiation and extirpation of the tumor.[6,19] Surgery has questionable benefits for those patients with nasal cavity adenocarcinoma.

MINIMALLY INVASIVE APPROACH

Small rigid endoscopes can be used to visualize contents of the nasal cavity. In addition, a diode laser can also be used to remove the nasal turbinates and tumor. Typically rigid endoscopes are used having a 2.7-mm diameter and a 30-degree angle at the tip. The 30-degree scope allows visualization around corners; however, this is usually not needed for most of the regions of the nasal cavity. One liter of lactated Ringer fluid spiked with 25 mL of 2% lidocaine with epinephrine (generally 1:100,000 epinephrine is used) is infused into the nasal cavity.[11,12] This technique decreases bleeding, clears the visual field of blood and debris, and reduces pain during the procedure.

COMPLICATIONS

In the immediate postoperative period, the patient's head should be slightly lowered to prevent aspiration of blood or remaining flush solution.[20,21] Continue to monitor the patient for signs of coughing, hypoxia, changes in lung sounds, and pattern of breathing because these are potential signs that aspiration has occurred. Patients with any clinical signs suggestive of aspiration pneumonia should undergo further diagnostic work-up and treatment. Excessive hemorrhage and anemia are possible. Roll gauze or umbilical tape can be packed in the caudal nasal cavity to adequately provide pressure to reduce bleeding. Another option is impregnation of gauze with petrolatum, which may reduce adhesion formation.[20] The packing material can stay in place for 24 hours after surgery and then be easily removed. Postoperative anemia, if severe, necessitates blood transfusions. Chronic recurrent secondary bacterial infection of the nasal cavity may occur and requires intermittent antibiotic therapy. Furthermore, secondary fungal infections or fungal hypersensitivity may develop because of a breakdown of normal defense mechanisms and may require infusion of the nasal cavity with clotrimazole cream. Extensive subcutaneous emphysema over the cranial or even the entire body is a common postoperative complication and is caused by air forced beneath the skin during sneezing. The

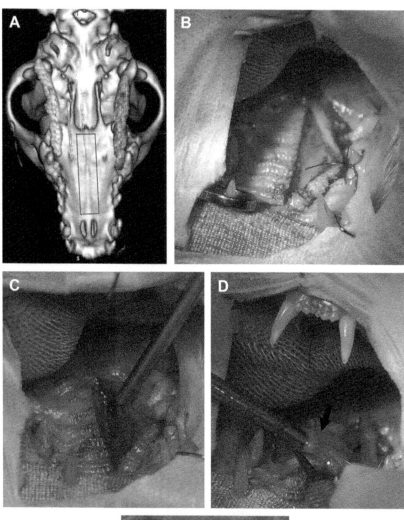

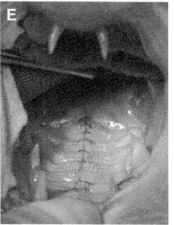

authors find that this complication is eliminated by providing a large temporary "blow hole" over the dorsal rhinotomy site during the first week after surgery. If an animal has an underdeveloped basilar arterial system, severe ischemic injury to the brain can occur if temporary carotid occlusion has been used during the procedure; this complication is more apt to occur in cats. Neurologic signs may also be seen if brain injury occurs following penetration of the ethmoidal turbinates. Bacterial menigoencephalitis is also a potential complication if the ethmoidal turbinates and meninges have been violated.

POSTOPERATIVE CARE

Eating must be encouraged in patients undergoing intranasal surgery and ablation of the turbinates. Sense of smell may be diminished, thereby leading to decreased appetite. Warm odiferous foods should be offered to encourage eating. It may be essential to syringe feed the patient or provide nutritional support via an esophagostomy or endoscopically placed gastrostomy tube. Administration of intravenous fluids may be needed for 1 or 2 days to maintain normal hydration and replace fluid losses associated with intraoperative bleeding. Dried blood and crusts that typically build up at the external nares must be removed to maintain a patent airway. If a "blow hole" has been left open over the dorsal rhinotomy, discharge and blood should be cleansed from this area to ensure patency during the first week after surgery. This hole heals quickly. If needed, a suture or staple can be placed to close the "blow hole," but this is typically not needed. Serosanguinous discharge from the external nares is present during the first week after surgery and this is normal in the postoperative period. A broad-spectrum antibiotic effective against bacteria that are found in the nasal cavity should be administered for a period of 2 weeks. If an intraoral procedure has been performed, soft food should be administered for a period of 2 weeks or until the incision has healed. Chew toys must be avoided during the healing phase.[9,11,14,15]

OUTCOMES

Recurrence of a malignant tumor is expected in most cases and clinical signs may recur within 6 to 12 months after surgery.[9,11,14,15,20] Rostrally located tumors respond more favorably to radiation therapy versus those that are in the area of the ethmoid turbinates. (For more information on feline nasopharyngeal polyps, see Greci V, Mortellaro CM: Management of Otic and Nasopharyngeal, and Nasal Polyps in Cats and Dogs, in this issue.)

◀────────────────────────────────────

Fig. 7. (A) Canine skull, ventral view. Three-dimensional CT reconstruction. Ventral rhinotomy proposed location delineated by the *rectangle*. (B) Domestic shorthair, 15-year-old female spayed. See **Fig. 5** for CT images of this case. A midline mucoperiosteal incision is made along the entire length of the hard palate to provide adequate exposure to the palatine bones. This image taken intraoperatively illustrates the use of stay sutures, placed on the elevated mucoperiosteal flap, providing retraction for better visualization of the underlying bone. (C) After the mucoperiosteum has been elevated from the hard palate, a fine rongeur is used to create a window in the palatine bone to complete the ventral approach. (D) This image taken intraoperatively illustrates extraction of the nasal polyp (*arrow*). (E) Closure of the mucoperiosteum is secured in one layer. The image depicts a closure of the mucoperiosteum using a simple interrupted suture pattern with the knots buried. Sutures are strategically placed in the valleys of the mucosal folds of the hard palate.

REFERENCES

1. Evans HE, editor. Miller's anatomy of the dog. 3rd edition. Philadelphia: Saunders; 1993. p. 463–72.
2. Evans HE, De Lahunta A. Guide to the dissection of the dog. 7th edition. Philadelphia: Saunders Elsevier; 2010. p. 221–55.
3. Madewell BR, Priester WA, Gillette EL, et al. Neoplasms of the nasal passages and paranasal sinuses in domesticated animals as reported by 13 veterinary colleges. Am J Vet Res 1976;37(7):851–6.
4. Ogilvie GK, LaRue SM. Canine and feline nasal and paranasal sinus tumors. Vet Clin North Am Small Anim Pract 1992;22(5):1133–44.
5. Lana SE, Turek MM. Tumors of the respiratory system: nasosinal tumors. In: Withrow SJ, MacEwen EG, editors. Small animal clinical oncology. 5th edition. Philadelphia: Saunders; 2013. p. 435–47.
6. Adams WM, Withrow SJ, Walshaw R, et al. Radiotherapy of malignant nasal tumors in 67 dogs. J Am Vet Med Assoc 1987;191:311–5.
7. Northrup NC, Etue SM, Ruslander DM, et al. Retrospective study of orthovoltage radiation therapy for nasal tumors in 42 dogs. J Vet Intern Med 2001; 15(3):183–9.
8. Adams WM, Bjorling DE, McAnalty JE, et al. Outcome of accelerated radiotherapy followed by extenteration of the nasal cavity in dogs with intranasal neoplasia: 53 cases (1990-2002). J Am Vet Med Assoc 2005;227(6):936–41.
9. Birchard SJ. Surgical diseases of the nasal cavity and paranasal sinuses. Semin Vet Med Surg (Small Anim) 1995;10(2):77–86.
10. Drees LR, Forrest LJ, Chappell R. Comparison of computed tomography and magnetic resonance imaging for the evaluation of canine intranasal neoplasia. J Small Anim Pract 2009;50(7):334–40.
11. Nelson WA. Nasal passages, sinus, and palate. In: Slatter D, editor. Textbook of small animal surgery, vol. 1, 3rd edition. Philadelphia: Saunders; 2003. p. 824–37.
12. Bojrab MJ. Current techniques in small animal surgery. 3rd edition. Philadelphia: Lea & Febiger; 1990. p. 321–6.
13. Hedlund CS, Tangner CH, Elkins AD, et al. Temporary bilateral carotid artery occlusion during surgical explorations of the nasal cavity in the dog. Vet Surg 1983; 12(2):83–6.
14. Holmberg DL, Fries C, Cockshutt J. Ventral rhinotomy in the dog and cat. Vet Surg 1989;18(6):446–9.
15. Holmberg DL. Sequelae of ventral rhinotomy in dogs and cats with inflammatory and neoplastic nasal pathology: a retrospective study. Can Vet J 1996;37:483–5.
16. Ter Haar G, Hampel R. Combined rostrolateral rhinotomy for removal of rostral nasal septum squamous cell carcinoma: long-term outcome in 10 dogs. Vet Surg 2015;44(7):843–51.
17. Pavletic MM. Nasal reconstruction techniques. In: Pavletic MM, editor. Atlas of small animal wound management and reconstructive surgery. 3rd edition. Ames (IA): Wiley-Blackwell; 2010. p. 573–602.
18. Mouatt JG, Straw RC. Use of mandibular symphysiotomy to allow extensive caudal hemimaxillectomy in a dog. Aust Vet J 2002;80(5):272–6.
19. Sones E, Smith A, Schiles S, et al. Survival times for canine intranasal sarcomas treated with radiation therapy: 86 cases (1996-2011). Vet Radiol Ultrasound 2013; 54(2):194–201.

20. Schmiedt CW, Creevy KE. Nasal planum, nasal cavity and sinuses. In: Tobias KM, Johnston SA, editors. Veterinary surgery: small animal. 1st edition. Philadelphia: Saunders; 2012. p. 1702–6.
21. Malinowski C. Canine and feline nasal neoplasia. Clin Tech Small Anim Pract 2006;21:89–94.

Nose and Nasal Planum Neoplasia, Reconstruction

Deanna R. Worley, DVM

KEYWORDS

- Intranasal lesions • Computed tomography • Nasal planectomy
- Radical planectomy

KEY POINTS

- Most intranasal lesions are best treated with radiation therapy.
- Computed tomographic imaging with intravenous contrast is critical for treatment planning.
- Computed tomographic images of the nose will best assess the integrity of the cribriform plate for central nervous system invasion by a nasal tumor.
- Because of an owner's emotional response to an altered appearance of their dog's face, discussions need to include the entire family before proceeding with nasal planectomy or radical planectomy.
- With careful case selection, nasal planectomy and radical planectomy surgeries can be locally curative.

DIAGNOSIS

Obtaining a diagnosis, whether cytologically or preferably histologically, precludes therapeutic intervention of the nose and nasal planum. Just as the eyes are perceived as windows to the soul, so also is the unaltered appearance of a pet's face. A variety of ablative procedures can be done to remove neoplastic lesions of the nose and nasal planum, and many are associated with disfigurement.

A nasal tumor should be on the list of differential diagnoses when dogs present with clinical signs ranging from crusting and/or a nonhealing ulcer on the nasal planum, to deformation of the nasal planum and nose. Unilateral or bilateral nasal discharge whether serous, mucoid, mucopurulent, or epistaxis is common for intranasal lesions. Ocular discharge may also result with obstruction of the nasolacrimal duct from a nasal tumor. The patient may show sensitivity during direct palpation of the nose and face, or palpable bony defects may be detectable. Dogs with intranasal obstruction from an intranasal mass may show severe distress when the mouth is held closed by an examiner during physical examination or during restraint. Similarly, sleeping

The author has nothing to disclose.
Surgical Oncology, Department of Clinical Sciences and Flint Animal Cancer Center, Colorado State University, 300 West Drake Road, Fort Collins, CO 80523, USA
E-mail address: deanna.worley@colostate.edu

difficulties, ranging from restlessness to disrupted sleep, arise from neoplastic obstruction of the nasal passage because some dogs will not adapt to open-mouth breathing even at rest.

Intranasal obstruction can be determined during physical examination from 3 different tests, perhaps the most reliable being a slide condensation test. A clean glass slide is held underneath the nares, and a normal result is the presence of 2 symmetric condensation patterns on the glossy slide. A wisp of cotton from a cotton ball is dangled in front of each nare and should wiggle with expiration. The more unpleasant test uses an examiner's finger placed over each nare, effectively blocking the unilateral passageway and detecting air movement from the unoccluded nare.

In the dog, the nasal planum is biopsied either with an incisional wedge biopsy or via a punch biopsy instrument. Because there is robust blood supply to the nose, these biopsy sites are best sutured closed to control hemorrhage. Intranasal biopsies are oftentimes obtained after advanced imaging, specifically a skull CT with contrast or endoscopically during rhinoscopy.[1] Endoscopic biopsies are small and may not always penetrate deep enough for a diagnostically representative sample. Conversely, retroflexed endoscopic biopsies from the choanae can be rewarding and are minimally invasive. With larger lesions present within the nasopharynx, rostral traction of the soft palate using a spay hook instrument can augment visualization for an incisional biopsy. Computed tomographic (CT) imaging of the nose and head with intravenous (IV) contrast greatly aids in diagnosis of potential lesions and in directing biopsy approach. Specific features seen on CT that are correlative of a nasal neoplasia include unilateral lysis of maxilla (dorsal and lateral), ethmoturbinates, and any lysis of the vomer bone, orbital lamina, and ventral maxilla.[2]

CT images of the nose will best assess the integrity of the cribriform plate for central nervous system (CNS) invasion by a tumor. It is important to note this because, if present, intranasal biopsy via hydropropulsion is contraindicated (**Fig. 1**). When the cribriform plate is intact, the hydropropulsion biopsy technique is a less hemorrhagic option that also results in temporary palliation by dislodging and removing chunks

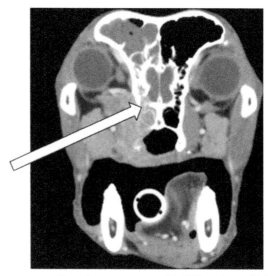

Fig. 1. Sinonasal squamous cell carcinoma as seen with CT imaging, which also reveals focal cribriform plate lysis (*white arrow*). Facial asymmetry was not detected.

of obstructing tumor tissue.[3] To perform this biopsy option, the patient is anesthetized with a securely inflated endotracheal tube. The nose is directed ventrally; one nare is occluded and either a 60-mL catheter tip syringe or large bulb syringe is lodged in the opposite nare. A large volume of saline is instilled forcibly antegrade into the nose. Loosened tumor samples and saline effluent travel through the nasopharynx and are collected orally as the patient's mouth is held open over a collecting basin. CT-acquired images, critical for targeted radiation planning purposes, also are essential in guiding best yield representative intranasal biopsies. Traumatic nasal biopsy techniques are quite bloody so preoperative blood typing, platelet count, coagulation testing, and blood pressure screening are advised before the procedure. Traumatic nasal biopsies are collected with a straw (typically the sterile sheath covering a spinal needle), with a bone curette, or some sort of biopsy forceps (uterine biopsy instrument, laryngeal cup forceps, alligator forceps). Any one of these instruments is inserted intranasally through the ventral meatus first after being premeasured to the medial canthus of the dog's eye. Instruments penetrating antegrate in a posterior direction are at risk of CNS biopsy at a depth past the medial canthus. The nose bleeds profusely following traumatic intranasal biopsies (less notably via the hydropropulsion technique), and most patients are able to be discharged as outpatient procedures. Epistaxis following traumatic nasal biopsy typically subsides in patients without further intervention, although use of ice packs may palliate.

Most nasal planum lesions, specifically solar-induced squamous cell carcinomas, occurring commonly in the cat, are superficial and appear as crusting and nonhealing superficial ulcers (**Fig. 2**). These lesions may also occur at the pinnae, palpebral margins, and area between the ears and eyes. Sometimes an impression smear results in a cytologic diagnosis. The more reliable means for diagnosis is with an incisional biopsy with a scalpel blade or with a small punch biopsy instrument.

CLINICAL MANAGEMENT
Sinonasal Carcinoma: Canine

Approximately two-thirds of neoplastic intranasal lesions occurring in the dog will be a carcinoma. The treatment of choice for sinonasal carcinomas is radiation therapy as a

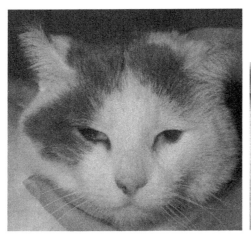
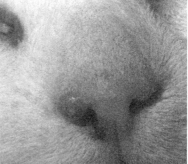

Fig. 2. Typical appearance of feline nasal planum squamous cell carcinoma characterized by superficial ulceration and crusting.

single modality or combined with cytoreductive surgery (and the reported median survival times [MSTs] range from 7 to 47 months, 15 months MST).[4–11] MSTs for dogs with nasal carcinomas not receiving treatment or receiving palliative treatment was 3 months, and cause of death or euthanasia was due to progressive local disease (and epistaxis was associated with shorter survival times in one report).[12] Similarly, the more common cause of death or euthanasia with curative-intent therapies was due to local tumor recurrence and less often from metastatic disease in another retrospective study.[13]

Nasal Planum Squamous Cell Carcinoma: Canine

Squamous cell carcinoma of the nasal planum in dogs tends to be more locally invasive than in cats. The biologic behavior of metastasis is slow, affecting local lymph nodes first.[14] Distant metastasis is possible, although most dogs are euthanized because of clinical signs of tumor recurrence, particularly following incomplete local tumor excision, before progression of distant metastasis.[14,15] In the dog nasal planum, squamous cell carcinomas are more successfully treated by local wide excision, although other less durable options exist, such as radiation therapy.[15] A local cure may also be possible following wide local excision. A challenge with wide excision of nasal planum squamous cell carcinoma in the dog is the difficulty in accurately determining the extent of the disease, because this can be very difficult to assess even with IV contrast-enhanced CT imaging, particularly at the level of the nasal conchae.[15,16] There is the possibility for improved assessment of extent of local disease with PET CT imaging.[17] Radiation therapy, piroxicam, and carboplatin do play a role in palliation therapy for nasal planum squamous cell carcinoma.[14,18,19]

Lymphoma

Nasal lymphoma is the more common nasal tumor in the cat.[20] Other common nasal tumor types in the cat include adenocarcinomas, squamous cell carcinomas, anaplastic carcinoma, and fibrosarcomas.[20] As in the dog, most intranasal tumors are more effectively managed with radiation therapy versus debulking procedures.[21] In one study, survival times ranged from 4 to 55 months, including complete remission, for cats receiving radiation therapy for stage I (single extranodal tumor) nasal lymphoma.[22] In another study, the median progression-free interval was 31 months.[23] Concurrent feline leukemia viral infection is uncommon with nasal lymphoma.[24]

Mast Cell Tumor

Mast cell tumors occurring on the muzzle behave more aggressively in this location than on other sites in the dog.[13] Normal anatomy constraints impact options for wide local excision in this region. However, incomplete excision of mast cell tumors occurring at the nose adversely impacts patient survival. Because mast cell tumors occurring on the muzzle behave more aggressively, are characterized by local infiltration, and are more commonly biologically high-grade mast cell tumors, accurate assessment of neoplastic infiltration in local regional lymph nodes is critical. As the lymphatic drainage of the nose is complex, the more accurate method for determining the at-risk lymph node or nodes receiving draining tumor lymph, and hence metastasis by migrating tumor cells, is with sentinel lymph node mapping.[25] Sentinel lymph node mapping can be performed using a combination of regional lymphoscintigraphy with technetium and intraoperative methylene blue dye, or anecdotally with indirect lymphography. A sentinel lymph node or nodes that are identified are extirpated to assess for histologic evidence of lymphatic metastasis. Removal of these nodes may also improve patient survival if positive for metastasis when node extirpation is combined with adjuvant curative-intent therapy, such as vinblastine and prednisone chemotherapy. During surgery, extirpation of sentinel lymph nodes precedes definitive tumor removal because the nose is a less clean surgical region. The ideal surgical margin to excise around a mast cell tumor of the muzzle remains unknown, and anatomic constraints limit the desired surgical margin. Grading information obtained from an incisional biopsy of a muzzle mast cell tumor combined with additional patient staging results, including regional lymph node status, optimizes the patient plan and surgical dose devised for each patient. Currently, 1-cm or greater margins are suggested for smaller breed dogs, and at least 1-cm but preferably 2- to 3-cm margins should be planned in larger dogs, because muzzle mast cell tumors are typically high grade. Alternatively, the diameter of the mast cell tumor may be used for determination of the surgical margin.[26] Morbidity may be mitigated after nasal surgery, especially following incomplete excision, with less assertive surgical excision combined with neoadjuvant radiation therapy and/or administration of neoadjuvant chemotherapy before embarking on a less aggressive local tumor excision option.

Sarcomas

Many sarcoma tumor types also occur in the nasal tissues, and within the nose and sinuses. These sarcomas include osteosarcoma, chondrosarcoma, and fibrosarcoma. Discussion of these tumor types are covered elsewhere in this issue (See Weeden AM, Degner DA: Surgical Approaches to the Nasal Cavity and Sinuses, in this issue.) It is important to note the awareness of histologically low-grade biologically high-grade fibrosarcomas in dogs, especially in the retriever breeds, as these can be misdiagnosed as benign processes such as fibroplasia or fibroma on histologic evaluation of incisional biopsy samples.

Surgical Options

"If tumor is touching bone, bone has to go..."

Clinical goals dictate clinical management, and clinical goals depend on decisions arising from the veterinarian-client partnership. Most intranasal lesions are best treated with radiation therapy, and risk of acute and late radiation side effects is mitigated with incorporation of 3-dimensional (3D) conformal radiation therapy, intensity-modulated radiation therapy, and stereotactic radiation therapy modalities[23] (**Fig. 3**). For lesions occurring on the surface of the nose, anatomic constraints and the desired surgical margin for a specific tumor type impact decision-making. Several questions should be asked before embarking on nasal mass excision with the intent for a local cure. Specific guidelines for surgical extirpation of nasal tumors remain unknown. What are the recommended surgical margin goals? Is it 0.5-cm, 1-cm, 2-cm resection away from the tumor? Is it the same for a small breed dog versus large breed dog? Should it include an uninvolved fascial plane beyond the tumor? Further uncertainty exists as to what are the ideal histologic margins to predict local cure for each unique tumor type, whether tumor cells are simply not touching the surgical edge,[27] whether tumor cells are seen less than 1 mm of the surgical edge, or are seen greater than 2 mm from the surgical margin. Planned surgical margins will not always equate with achieved histologic margins, so both are factored into presurgical planning and for adjuvant therapy considerations.

Superficial lesions less than 2 mm in thickness may be treated with cryotherapy; typically this is recommended in cats with superficial squamous cell carcinoma lesions

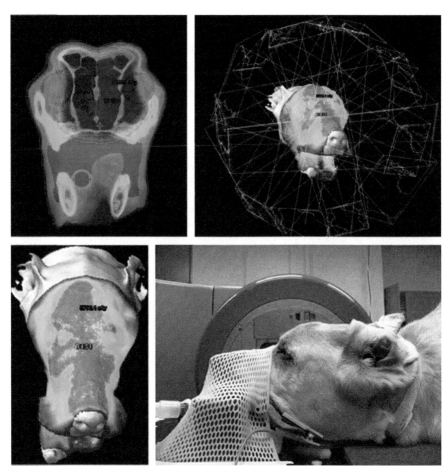

Fig. 3. Most sinonasal tumors are best treated with radiation therapy because great advances have been made in limiting patient morbidity particularly because the acute and late radiation side effects have been mitigated through incorporation of 3D conformal radiation therapy, intensity-modulated radiation therapy, and stereotactic radiation therapy modalities.

(**Fig. 4**). Cryotherapy is followed with active surveillance and serial cryotherapy treatments for any new superficial lesions, whether done monthly, every 6 months, or annually, depending on whether there is progression of lesions. There is a plethora of other options reported for treatment of superficial squamous cell carcinoma, including topical retinoids, photodynamic therapy, strontium (Sr 90), and electrochemotherapy.[28,29]

Nasal planecotomies are best suited for invasive lesions within the nasal planum, and not extending caudally into the nasal conchae. After excision of the nasal planum, the defect is sutured closed with loose reapposition of the skin to the nasal mucosa, and/or soft tissues are secured with suture to the exposed bone using bone tunnels (**Figs. 5–7**).

For tumors characterized by locoregional lymph node metastasis, regional metastatic and/or sentinel lymph nodes are extirpated as part of tumor management,

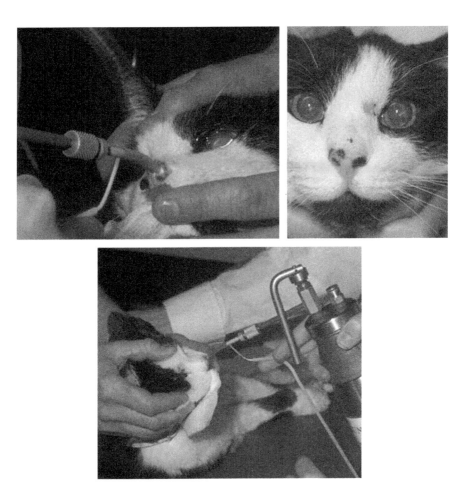

Fig. 4. Cryotherapy is an effective tool for managing nasal planar superficial solar-induced squamous cell carcinoma lesions in the cat. Demonstrated here, 2 cycles of a rapid freeze slow thaw via probe application cryotherapy resulted in effective posttreatment eschars.

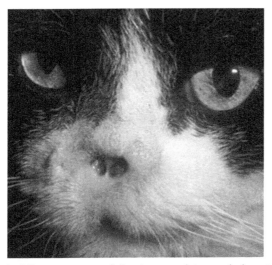

Fig. 5. Characteristic feline appearance following complete nasal planectomy surgery.

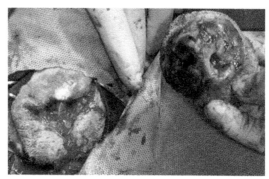

Fig. 6. Intraoperative appearance of canine nasal planectomy surgery without maxillectomy. Left, completed repair; right, excised nasal planum.

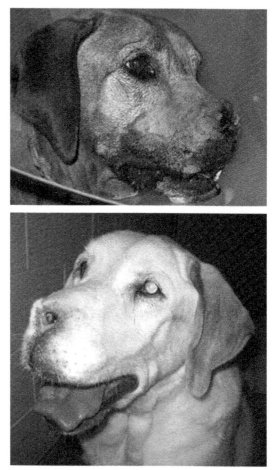

Fig. 7. Characteristic canine appearance following nasal planectomy surgery without maxillectomy.

particularly if combined with primary tumor removal and if removal will impact adjuvant therapy decision-making and/or patient survival.

For invasive lesions penetrating deeper than the nasal planum, extending caudally into the premaxilla/maxilla or nasal conchae, a combined approach of bilateral rostral maxillectomy and nasal planectomy is recommended.[30] CT imaging with IV contrast is critical for surgical planning as well as thorough presurgical counseling due to a drastically altered patient facial appearance. The patient is positioned sternally, and the mouth is held partially opened with a gag. The pharynx is packed with a sponge to prevent hemorrhage from draining into the airways. When using a hanging mouth position for surgery, try to maintain full mobility of the labium to aid in the reconstruction and closure. In addition, use of a sterile marking pen and ruler helps in achieving the desired planned surgical margin because tissues will become distorted during retraction and resection. Expect the nose and muzzle to bleed profusely during the procedure. Electrocautery (caution with application of this modality on mucosal surfaces) and vascular clips, particularly on palatine and sphenopalatine arteries, help reduce bleeding. The depth of caudal resection will vary on the breed of dog, location of tumor, and surgical margin desired for a planned complete resection. However, the recommended caudal limit for bilateral maxillectomy is just caudal to either second or third premolar tooth for most patients. Dissection progresses from skin excision to the subcutaneous and nasolabial muscular layers to the bone. Bilateral maxillectomy resection with an oscillating saw completes the combined en-bloc resection (**Fig. 8**). To accurately assess surgical margins histologically, tissue marking dyes are applied to the ex vivo specimen.

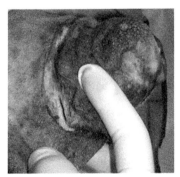
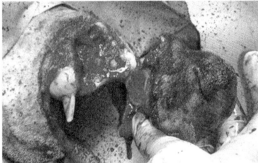
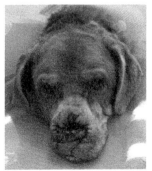

Fig. 8. Intraoperative resection of an extensive nasal planum fibrosarcoma requiring bilateral rostral maxillectomy and nasal planectomy procedure and patient appearance 1 day postoperatively.

The most technically challenging part of aggressive planectomy and rostral maxillectomy lies in reconstruction of the defect.[31,32] Options include bilateral labial mucocutaneous advancement flaps created from incisions of the labiogingival border (caution to not extend the incision too far caudally at the level of the commissure because this may interrupt vascular supply via angularis oris artery), bilateral buccal mucocutaneous rotation-advancement flaps, purse-string closure, some variation of a unilateral labial mucocutaneous advancement flap, or even possibly a transposition flap of nasal skin in dogs possessing redundant nasal skin folds.[30,32–34] A practical tip is to restore the mucosal layer first between the labium and palate. Use of bone tunnels created by drilling a Kirschner wire into the palatine and frontal bones helps to secure labial submucosa, muscle, and dermis and may help obtain tension-free apposition of the wound. When possible, skin should be apposed to the nasal mucosa (**Fig. 9**).

Controversies and Complications

Obtaining a cosmetic facial appearance is perhaps the greatest challenge following nasal planectomy and radical planectomy, and this is an important consideration to discuss with the owner before surgery. Because of the emotional response owners have to an altered facial appearance on their pet after nasal surgery, the entire family unit should be included on the decision. Representative images of dogs and cats with similar nasal surgeries should be shown to owners to prepare them for this concern. Even with thorough preoperative client education, the postoperative facial appearance following resection can be highly disturbing to owners. Unprepared owners have been known to alienate their pet at home and avoid petting and cuddling. Likewise, they can be unprepared to deal with interactions of unversed strangers and their dogs during walks. The altered facial appearance after nasal surgery can be mistaken by unfamiliar dogs as an aggressive expression, so the author cautions owners to avoid intermingling with unfamiliar dogs.

Healing challenges persist following nasal planectomy and radical planectomy. Dogs will persistently lick their nose following nasal surgery, and this may disrupt

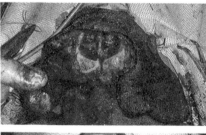
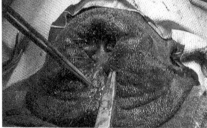
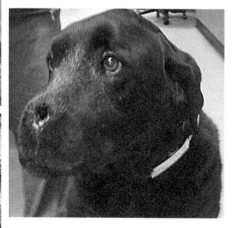

Fig. 9. Intraoperative resection of an extensive nasal planum fibrosarcoma requiring bilateral rostral maxillectomy and nasal planectomy procedure and patient appearance months postoperatively.

the delicate skin to mucosa suture line directly overlying the ostectomized bone (**Fig. 10**). When dehiscence occurs, especially with resulting bony exposure, immediate or delayed primary reclosure is the goal. As the nose is well vascularized, surgical site infection contributes secondarily to dehiscence and exacerbates dehiscence but rarely is the sole cause of dehiscence, unlike traumatic causes. Dehiscence risk is reduced by limiting other forms of self-trauma with restrictive Elizabethan collars and/or, rarely, hobbles. In addition, providing soft or liquefied foods, and avoiding dry kibble or any other hard chew objects for 3 to 4 weeks, may also protect the healing wound. Dehiscence needs to be avoided because it can also result in oronasal fistula formation and an exposed dental arcade.

Another particular challenge of nasal surgery is avoiding the risk of nasal orifice stenosis or cicatrix, which can occur as early as 2 weeks postoperatively (**Fig. 11**). As the

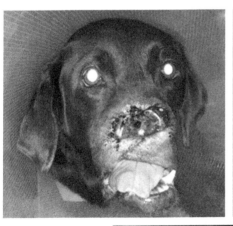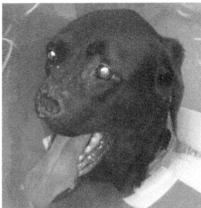

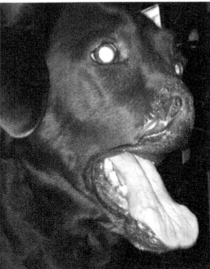

Fig. 10. Labrador retriever demonstrating postoperative radical planectomy incisional dehiscence secondary to licking by the dog's tongue, with 1-week and 6-month appearance following primary closure revision surgery.

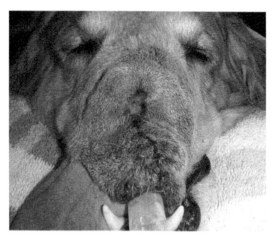

Fig. 11. Appearance of nasal orifice stenosis or cicatrix formation 1 month following combined bilateral rostral maxillectomy and nasal planectomy. The right orifice was completely obliterated by scar tissue and the left had a 2-mm-diameter patent ostium.

surgical site heals, the patient is also prone to nasal bleeding (typically for about a week), nasal crusting, and ulceration (**Fig. 12**). Persistent crusting and superficial ulceration may contribute to cicatrix formation, but disruption in mucosal apposition is of most concern. The use of a variety of intranasal stents to reduce recurrent cicatrix formation in dogs following nasal planectomy surgery has been anecdotally described, but

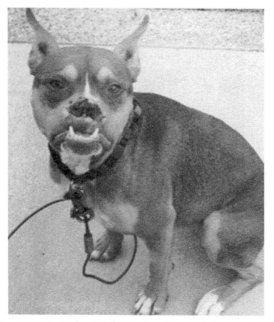

Fig. 12. Temporary crusting and superficial ulceration of the nasal orifice is expected following radical planectomy surgery.

efficacy is not established. Direct application of mitomycin C has also be anecdotally described for treatment of recurrent cicatrix formation, and efficacy is not established. Sharp excision of stenotic cicatrix occluding the nasal orifice with loose reapposition of skin anecdotally is not a therapeutic solution because recurrent cicatrix will result. Surgical reconstruction should aim to best reappose intranasal or well-vascularized mucosa to skin. Most animals will not be amenable to regular postoperative saline irrigation of the nasal planectomy site to limit secondary nasal crusting. Translational review of human choanal atresia repair experiences and of cicatrix formation reveals that use of postoperative intraluminal stents failed to show in meta-analysis a difference in surgical outcome of choanal atresia repair.[35] In addition, the use of mitomycin C as an adjunct for human surgical choanal atresia repair is currently not supported.[35] It has also been found in humans with transnasal endoscopic repair of choanal atresia that postoperative restenosis is prevented with complete covering of exposed bony surfaces with mucosa, and frequent postoperative nasal saline irrigation and removal of nasal crusting a week after the primary repair reduce the rate of restenosis.[35]

With advanced sinonasal neoplasms, progressive and acute epistaxis can be a life-threatening risk. Palliation can include unilateral or bilateral carotid artery ligation to reduce arterial supply to the nose. In the cat, the arterial circle of the brain is incomplete with predominant brain blood supply derived from branches of the external carotid arteries. Therefore, only unilateral carotid arterial ligation should be considered in this species.[36] More precise reduction of tumor-associated epistaxis may be achieved with selective arterial embolization with interventional radiology.[37]

For large and difficult sinonasal fistulae, including loss of the nasal planum, resulting as a sequelae to surgical and/or radiation therapies, an indirect distant bipedicle subdermal plexus flap, or tube flap, may be considered for reconstruction (Laurent Findji and Richard Walshaw, personal communication, 2015). The length-to-width ratio for development of the tube flap should not exceed 6–8x by 1x in size, and it may take 6 to 8 weeks

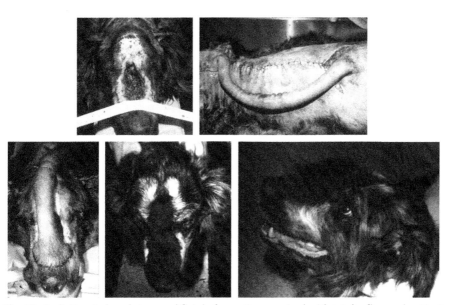

Fig. 13. Radiation-induced sinonasal fistula formation repaired with a tube flap and patient appearance following delayed flap division and wound healing. (*Courtesy of* Richard Walshaw, BVMS, DACVS, Dearborn, MI, USA.)

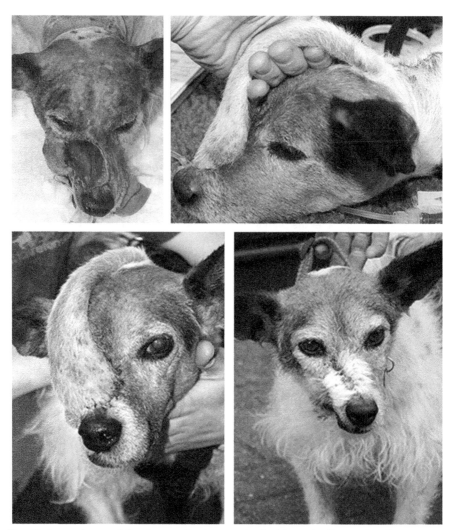

Fig. 14. Large sinonasal fistula complication repaired with a tube flap and patient appearance following delayed flap division and wound healing. (*Courtesy of* Laurent Findji, DMV, MS, MRCVS, DECVS, Laindon, Essex, UK.)

for complete transfer to the recipient site (**Figs. 13** and **14**). Historically, Heinrick von Pfalzpaint in 1460 reconstructed traumatically avulsed human noses in Europe using a skin flap from the upper arm, which was sutured to the nasal defect and with the arm bandaged to the head before flap division 8 to 10 days later.[38] Even more ancient, use of a forehead tubed flap for human nasal avulsions was described in India as early as ~700 BC and is currently a gold standard for human nasal reconstructions.[39]

REFERENCES

1. Finck M, Ponce F, Guilbaud L, et al. Computed tomography or rhinoscopy as the first-line procedure for suspected nasal tumor: a pilot study. Can Vet J 2015; 56(2):185–92.

2. Tromblee TC, Jones JC, Etue AE, et al. Association between clinical characteristics, computed tomography characteristics, and histologic diagnosis for cats with sinonasal disease. Vet Radiol Ultrasound 2006;47(3):241–8.

3. Day MJ, Henderson SM, Belshaw Z, et al. An immunohistochemical investigation of 18 cases of feline nasal lymphoma. J Comp Pathol 2004;130(2–3):152–61.

4. Theon AP, Madewell BR, Harb MF, et al. Megavoltage irradiation of neoplasms of the nasal and paranasal cavities in 77 dogs. J Am Vet Med Assoc 1993;202(9):1469–75.

5. Henry CJ, Brewer WG Jr, Tyler JW, et al. Survival in dogs with nasal adenocarcinoma: 64 cases (1981-1995). J Vet Intern Med 1998;12(6):436–9.

6. LaDue TA, Dodge R, Page RL, et al. Factors influencing survival after radiotherapy of nasal tumors in 130 dogs. Vet Radiol Ultrasound 1999;40(3):312–7.

7. Northrup NC, Etue SM, Ruslander DM, et al. Retrospective study of orthovoltage radiation therapy for nasal tumors in 42 dogs. J Vet Intern Med 2001;15(3):183–9.

8. Adams WM, Bjorling DE, McAnulty JE, et al. Outcome of accelerated radiotherapy alone or accelerated radiotherapy followed by exenteration of the nasal cavity in dogs with intranasal neoplasia: 53 cases (1990-2002). J Am Vet Med Assoc 2005;227(6):936–41.

9. Adams WM, Miller PE, Vail DM, et al. An accelerated technique for irradiation of malignant canine nasal and paranasal sinus tumors. Vet Radiol Ultrasound 1998;39(5):475–81.

10. Bowles K, DeSandre-Robinson D, Kubicek L, et al. Outcome of definitive fractionated radiation followed by exenteration of the nasal cavity in dogs with sinonasal neoplasia: 16 cases. Vet Comp Oncol 2014. http://dx.doi.org/10.1111/vco.12115.

11. Lana SE, Dernell WS, Lafferty MH, et al. Use of radiation and a slow-release cisplatin formulation for treatment of canine nasal tumors. Vet Radiol Ultrasound 2004;45(6):577–81.

12. Rassnick KM, Goldkamp CE, Erb HN, et al. Evaluation of factors associated with survival in dogs with untreated nasal carcinomas: 139 cases (1993-2003). J Am Vet Med Assoc 2006;229(3):401–6.

13. Gieger TL, Theon AP, Werner JA, et al. Biologic behavior and prognostic factors for mast cell tumors of the canine muzzle: 24 cases (1990-2001). J Vet Intern Med 2003;17(5):687–92.

14. Lascelles BD, Parry AT, Stidworthy MF, et al. Squamous cell carcinoma of the nasal planum in 17 dogs. Vet Rec 2000;147(17):473–6.

15. Ter Haar G, Hampel R. Combined rostrolateral rhinotomy for removal of rostral nasal septum squamous cell carcinoma: long-term outcome in 10 dogs. Vet Surg 2015;44(7):843–51.

16. Adams WM, Kleiter MM, Thrall DE, et al. Prognostic significance of tumor histology and computed tomographic staging for radiation treatment response of canine nasal tumors. Vet Radiol Ultrasound 2009;50(3):330–5.

17. Yoshikawa H, Randall EK, Kraft SL, et al. Comparison between 2-(18) F-fluoro-2-deoxy-d-glucose positron emission tomography and contrast-enhanced computed tomography for measuring gross tumor volume in cats with oral squamous cell carcinoma. Vet Radiol Ultrasound 2013;54(3):307–13.

18. Langova V, Mutsaers AJ, Phillips B, et al. Treatment of eight dogs with nasal tumours with alternating doses of doxorubicin and carboplatin in conjunction with oral piroxicam. Aust Vet J 2004;82(11):676–80.

19. de Vos JP, Burm AG, Focker AP, et al. Piroxicam and carboplatin as a combination treatment of canine oral non-tonsillar squamous cell carcinoma: a pilot study and a literature review of a canine model of human head and neck squamous cell carcinoma. Vet Comp Oncol 2005;3(1):16–24.

20. Mukaratirwa S, van der Linde-Sipman JS, Gruys E. Feline nasal and paranasal sinus tumours: clinicopathological study, histomorphological description and diagnostic immunohistochemistry of 123 cases. J Feline Med Surg 2001;3(4): 235–45.

21. Henderson SM, Bradley K, Day MJ, et al. Investigation of nasal disease in the cat–a retrospective study of 77 cases. J Feline Med Surg 2004;6(4):245–57.

22. North SM, Meleo K, Mooney S, et al. Radiation therapy in the treatment of nasal lymphoma in cats. Proceedings of the 14th Annual Conference of the Veterinary Cancer Society. Townsend, TN; 1994. p. 21.

23. Sfiligoi G, Theon AP, Kent MS. Response of nineteen cats with nasal lymphoma to radiation therapy and chemotherapy. Vet Radiol Ultrasound 2007;48(4):388–93.

24. Moore A. Extranodal lymphoma in the cat: prognostic factors and treatment options. J Feline Med Surg 2013;15(5):379–90.

25. Worley DR. Incorporation of sentinel lymph node mapping in dogs with mast cell tumours: 20 consecutive procedures. Vet Comp Oncol 2014;12(3):215–26.

26. Pratschke KM, Atherton MJ, Sillito JA, et al. Evaluation of a modified proportional margins approach for surgical resection of mast cell tumors in dogs: 40 cases (2008-2012). J Am Vet Med Assoc 2013;243(10):1436–41.

27. Wittekind C, Compton C, Quirke P, et al. A uniform residual tumor (R) classification: integration of the R classification and the circumferential margin status. Cancer 2009;115(15):3483–8.

28. Spugnini EP, Vincenzi B, Citro G, et al. Electrochemotherapy for the treatment of squamous cell carcinoma in cats: a preliminary report. Vet J 2009;179(1):117–20.

29. Lucroy MD, Long KR, Blaik MA, et al. Photodynamic therapy for the treatment of intranasal tumors in 3 dogs and 1 cat. J Vet Intern Med 2003;17(5):727–9.

30. Lascelles BD, Henderson RA, Seguin B, et al. Bilateral rostral maxillectomy and nasal planectomy for large rostral maxillofacial neoplasms in six dogs and one cat. J Am Anim Hosp Assoc 2004;40(2):137–46.

31. Lascelles BD, Dernell WS, Correa MT, et al. Improved survival associated with postoperative wound infection in dogs treated with limb-salvage surgery for osteosarcoma. Ann Surg Oncol 2005;12(12):1073–83.

32. Gallegos J, Schmiedt CW, McAnulty JF. Cosmetic rostral nasal reconstruction after nasal planum and premaxilla resection: technique and results in two dogs. Vet Surg 2007;36(7):669–74.

33. Benlloch-Gonzalez M, Lafarge S, Bouvy B, et al. Nasal-skin-fold transposition flap for upper lip reconstruction in a French bulldog. Can Vet J 2013;54(10):983–6.

34. Yates G, Landon B, Edwards G. Investigation and clinical application of a novel axial pattern flap for nasal and facial reconstruction in the dog. Aust Vet J 2007; 85(3):113–8.

35. Kwong KM. Current updates on choanal atresia. Front Pediatr 2015;3:52.

36. Altay UM, Skerritt GC, Hilbe M, et al. Feline cerebrovascular disease: clinical and histopathologic findings in 16 cats. J Am Anim Hosp Assoc 2011;47(2):89–97.

37. Weisse C, Nicholson ME, Rollings C, et al. Use of percutaneous arterial embolization for treatment of intractable epistaxis in three dogs. J Am Vet Med Assoc 2004;224(8):1307–11, 281.

38. Greig A, Gohritz A, Geishauser M, et al. Heinrich von Pfalzpaint, pioneer of arm flap nasal reconstruction in 1460, more than a century before Tagliacozzi. J Craniofac Surg 2015;26(4):1165–8.

39. Correa BJ, Weathers WM, Wolfswinkel EM, et al. The forehead flap: the gold standard of nasal soft tissue reconstruction. Semin Plast Surg 2013;27(2):96–103.

Index

Note: Page numbers of article titles are **boldface** type.

A

Age
in cleft primary palate intervention, 666
Arytenoidectomy
partial
in laryngeal paralysis management, 711
Aural polyps
in dogs, 654
Auricular hematomas, **635–641**
introduction, 635
patient evaluation of, 636
recurrence of
prognosis for, 639–640
treatment of, **635–641**
nonpharmacologic, 636
options in, 636–639
pharmacologic, 636–637
postoperative care, 639
surgical, 637–639

B

Balloon dilation
in NPS management, 682–683
Bifid nose
repair of
in cleft primary palate reconstruction, 670–672
Bilateral cleft
repair of
in cleft primary palate reconstruction, 669
severe
repair of
in cleft primary palate reconstruction, 669–670
Brachycephalic syndrome (BS), **691–707**
anatomic and pathophysiologic changes in, 691–694
laryngeal, tracheal, and bronchial anomalies, 692–694
skull conformation anomalies, 691–692
soft tissue changes, 692
described, 691
diagnosis of, 694–695
gastroesophageal diseases associated with, 694
genesis of

Vet Clin Small Anim 46 (2016) 751–759
http://dx.doi.org/10.1016/S0195-5616(16)30009-2
0195-5616/16/$ – see front matter

Moving?

Make sure your subscription moves with you!

To notify us of your new address, find your **Clinics Account Number** (located on your mailing label above your name), and contact customer service at:

Email: journalscustomerservice-usa@elsevier.com

800-654-2452 (subscribers in the U.S. & Canada)
314-447-8871 (subscribers outside of the U.S. & Canada)

Fax number: 314-447-8029

Elsevier Health Sciences Division
Subscription Customer Service
3251 Riverport Lane
Maryland Heights, MO 63043

*To ensure uninterrupted delivery of your subscription, please notify us at least 4 weeks in advance of move.

Printed and bound by CPI Group (UK) Ltd, Croydon, CR0 4YY

03/10/2024

01040398-0016